Environmental Physiology

Environmental Physiology

D. BELLAMY D Phil
Professor of Zoology,
University College, Cardiff

G. J. GOLDSWORTHY Ph D
Lecturer in Zoology,
University of Hull

K. C. HIGHNAM Ph D
Reader in Zoology,
University of Sheffield

W. MORDUE Ph D
Senior Lecturer in Zoology,
Imperial College, London

J. G. PHILLIPS D Sc
Professor of Zoology,
University of Hull

EDITED BY J. G. PHILLIPS

A HALSTED PRESS BOOK

JOHN WILEY & SONS
NEW YORK

© 1975 Blackwell Scientific Publications
Osney Mead, Oxford
3 Nottingham Street, London W1M 3RA
9 Forrest Road, Edinburgh
P.O. Box 9, North Balwyn, Victoria, Australia

First published 1975

Published in the U.S.A. by Halsted Press,
a Division of John Wiley & Sons, Inc., New York

Library of Congress Cataloging in Publication Data

Phillips, J   G
      Environmental physiology.

      Includes index.
      1. Adaptation (Physiology)   I.   Bellamy, Denis.
II. Title.
QP82.P44   591.1   74-22107
ISBN 0-470-68490-9

Printed in Great Britain

Contents

Preface

All forms of animal life face to a greater or lesser degree environmental pressures which operate to displace an animal's physiological status from an 'ideal norm' or 'optimum'. The cushioning of a marine organism in a relatively unchanging environment, comparable in its constancy to that experienced by many internal parasites, and the severity of environment to which for example the desert and polar animals are subjected illustrate the possible extremes of such environmental pressures. Animals may react to restore the optimum physiological status through control mechanisms which reside at the cellular, tissue, organismal and behavioural levels. Their capacity to respond with adjustments to restore the 'norm' defines for each animal the limits for survival and dictates the organism's distribution within the many potential global habitats. The importance of the assessment of environmental factors in the physiology of animals has in recent years become increasingly clear and has brought closer together than ever before the interrelationship of two important biological disciplines of ecology and physiology. This book seeks to give expression to this conceptual link. It has been written with the two-fold purpose of providing on the one hand a basic text for a course in environmental physiology and on the other a comparative viewpoint to complement a more classical course in physiology; in so doing highlighting for the student the necessity of considering the impact of the environment on the evolving organism and conversely the effect of animals including man on their environments. Although the book is directed primarily at an undergraduate audience in University or Polytechnic Institutions, its emphasis on the conceptual approach stressing principles rather than detail will, it is hoped, prove a useful contribution to courses in Biology for Senior School Work and in Colleges of Further Education.

The authors wish to acknowledge permission to reproduce several figures in the text and reference is made in each case to the original publication.

Finally, we should like to record our very grateful thanks to Mrs. Barbara Taylor who patiently typed the various drafts of this book and to Dr. Judith Cheeseman for help in proof reading. Mr. Robert Campbell of Blackwell Scientific Publications Limited has at all times been helpful and co-operative during the preparation of this book and we wish to record our warm thanks for his assistance.

J. G. Phillips
Hull, 1974

TO
PROFESSOR IAN CHESTER-JONES

Part I
Basic Relationships with the Environment

Chapter 1
The External Environment
and the Whole Organism

Introduction

When cells are removed from the body and cultured under test-tube conditions they are very sensitive to slight changes in the composition of the culture medium. This fact is remarkable when it is realized that most intact animals are little affected by changes of a similar magnitude in the composition of their external environment. It is the aim of this book to reconcile this apparent paradox; the fact that cellular systems can only operate within a narrow range of external conditions, whereas whole animals are able to survive in widely differing environments. The situation for man, who may undergo brief exposure to dry heat which would boil water and still maintain a normal body temperature, illustrates this capacity of the whole body to withstand environmental change. Similarly, seals in the Arctic—under 30° of frost—have the same high body temperature as captive animals in British zoos. In desert areas, the resident animals and plants have no difficulty in retaining their body fluids in a hot dry atmosphere. These examples highlight the vast range of physical stresses to which animal life has become resistant. Temperatures endured by animal life cover a 60° range; pressures vary from a few pounds per square inch to several tons; the chemical composition of aquatic habitats covers over a hundred-fold concentration range. Whereas survival and growth of individuals is possible over a wide range of environmental conditions, propagation of species may require much narrower limits. For example, in the American oyster (*Ostrea virginica*) growth can occur between temperatures of 8 and 30°C while the capacities for reproduction has a very much narrower range of between 16 and 18°C.

Evolutionary aspects of environmental independence

All of these examples refer to a high degree of independence of external conditions. There is also a built-in resistance to internal changes that might otherwise prove disastrous to life. For instance, if the extra body heat produced by a long-distance runner was not rapidly dissipated by special methods, such as sweating and hyperventilation of the lungs, the rise in body temperature would be so great that some of the constituents of the body would become solid like a hard-boiled egg.

The perfection of mechanisms for holding a stable state in the face of extensive shifts in external environment is the consequence of gradual evolution of living things. In the millions of years during which animals have inhabited the earth they have tried many ways of protecting themselves against an unpredictable and varying world. The evolution of many groups of animals leads to a progressive independence of the environment. Frogs, for example, have not acquired the capacity to restrict evaporation of body water through the skin and when a frog leaves damp conditions it loses water, dries up and dies. Nor have frogs a means of keeping the temperature of the body above that of their surroundings. But frogs in their turn are capable of exploiting environments which are denied to most fish, apart from a few specialized species such as *Periopthalmus* (the mud skipper) which emerge from their aquatic environment and can respire in air; for fish in general require the relatively unchanged and cushioned environment of the seas or bodies of fresh water. Only a relatively few species, such as the Salmon or *Fundulus* (the killifish), are capable of free movement between fresh and sea water.

Slightly more advanced vertebrates, such as snakes, have developed a thick skin as a protection against water loss. They are therefore not confined to wet areas. However, like the frog, snakes are poikilotherms, that is animals whose temperature fluctuates with the environment, and during the winter, temperate species must hibernate as the environmental temperature is too low to maintain an active life.

Because of the many methods man has for combating the physical world, he is often regarded as the highest form of life on earth. However, this does not mean that man is better able to cope with extreme physical changes than other animals. For instance, certain birds, because they possess specialized mechanisms for salt excretion, can survive at sea by being able to use sea water for drinking purposes, whereas to man, who does not have these mechanisms, sea water, because of its high salt content, is toxic. Also, rats that live in deserts are able to survive on very dry food with no drinking water; man cannot do this. In order to explore seas and deserts, man must carry a supply of water and have shelter from the elements. Only by his foresight and his technology is man unique in being able to exploit every part of the earth. He owes this position as the most versatile form of life more to his advanced brain than to the possession of specific mechanisms for overcoming variations in the external world. Nevertheless, organisms—particularly man—continue to live and carry out their functions in a world that is subject to rapid and profound physical changes. This implies the existence of various internal systems which serve to maintain and restore the normal state against disturbing factors. The next section will be concerned with some of the regulatory devices which are generally employed by animals to keep the body in balance with the world outside.

Principles of homeostasis

The term 'homeostasis' is used to cover all the co-ordinated physiological processes by which each organism maintains itself in a steady state. This statement implies that organisms are able to 'perceive' an end point to which they adjust their activities. These activities are manifest at the organ, system, species and social levels, but ultimately there is a basic cellular reaction (or reactions) which underlies these adjustments. Thus, for all organisms, there are optimum conditions for life which at any point in time may be expressed in terms of the composition of the internal environment. We talk about regulatory mechanisms whereby organisms minimize the internal effects of environmental changes in, for example, temperature and salt content on the one hand, and population density on the other. The properties of the internal environment always change less than those of the external environment. However, the presence of homeostatic mechanisms does not imply a lack of change because the end point or value for the optimum steady state condition may shift with time.

The study of homeostatic mechanisms leads to an understanding of how different organisms are able to live and reproduce under adverse conditions. The term 'adverse' is used in the sense that *no* organism can maintain itself in *any* environment without effort. Problems of homeostasis are not so marked in a temperate climate as they are in polar or equatorial regions, but the problems encountered in the latter areas are merely temperate problems magnified many times, but in different environmental directions.

There are three theoretical ways in which homeostasis may be accomplished.
(1) If the environmental change is predictable, a timed device could provide a periodic internal counterpoise to the known fluctuation.
(2) The external conditions could be assessed and, together with a knowledge of the properties of the reacting system, an estimate could be made as to the extent of the anticipated change. An appropriate response could then be initiated to counteract the expected change.
(3) The internal condition could be monitored and any undue departure from a desirable norm could be used as a signal to initiate a response which would stop only when the norm had been restored.

Types of control systems in homeostasis

Of the three possible systems, only the first and third are utilized as biological mechanisms. The presence of the first mechanism in several physiological and biochemical activities is implicit in the existence of what are known as circadian rhythms. A circadian rhythm implies that a function occurs periodically with a periodicity of *about* 24 hours. Usually, circadian rhythms are synchronized with a 24-hour period by a cue from the external environment such as the time of sunrise or sunset (see Chapter 9).

Some of these rhythms anticipate a regular fluctuation in the external environment. For example, in nocturnal rodents, there is a continuous period of about twelve hours in each day during which the animal is asleep. This normally coincides with the daylight period. However, if rats are kept in continuous darkness, they still show this periodicity in sleep, indicating that an endogenous timing mechanism exists which regulates behaviour to fit the day length that has existed since they first evolved.

Although we know a great deal about circadian rhythms it is clear that animals are controlled by other endogenous rhythms of longer duration such as selenian cycles (about 28 days) and reproductive cycles which range in different species from four days to about a year. Although many of these cycles coincide with periodic changes in the physical environment, in the case of the circadian rhythms the environment often appears to be sharpening up an intrinsic rhythmical process.

The third kind of control system needs no internal clock or memory and works without information on the prevailing external conditions. The actual situation within the system is compared with the desired condition and appropriate action taken to correct any deficiency. This type of feedback system is known as a servo-mechanism and appears to be a most important arrangement by which organisms tolerate a changing environment. It is also of great importance in the automatic regulation of machines in the non-living world, and much of the terminology used to describe homeostasis in living things is taken from machine technology.

It is convenient to describe the servo-mechanisms of organisms first in relation to the environment change which triggers the homeostatic response. Changes in the environment may be of a physical, chemical or social nature and are ultimately detected as alterations in the chemical composition of the body. Chemical changes are the ultimate signals to which cells respond; a rise in temperature will increase the rate of a critical reaction; a change in the intensity or colour of light is translated into a new molecular configuration in the visual pigments through light-sensitive reactions; variations in the availability of food and water are monitored as changes in osmotic pressure or ionic composition of cells.

A change in the external environment may be restricted in its effect to a particular organ, for example, the eye, or it may produce a general change, such as osmotic pressure, that affects all cells. In the latter situation, only a restricted type of cell has the capacity to monitor the stimulus and transmit a signal to other specific cell types to initiate an appropriate response.

Analogy with servo-mechanisms

It is a characteristic of all servo-mechanisms that the overall response is a property of three distinct units which function together (Fig. 1.1). The central unit may be termed the controller which accepts the signal and interprets it. The signal comes into the controller from the detector and this signal may be termed the input stimulus. The controller is able to activate the appropriate response by means of an output stimulus to the third unit (the regulator), which responds to offset the change which initiated the input stimulus. The output of a homeo-static system is measured in terms of power or energy and the effect of the output

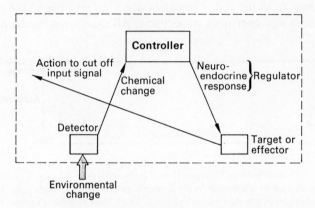

Figure 1.1. A basic servo-mechanism. (From D. Bellamy (1970) Animal rhythms. *Science Progress*, **58**, 99–115.)

is to reduce the input stimulus by restoring the system to normal. Looking at this three-point system as a whole, we can see that the original change has reacted back upon itself; a sequence of events occurs which neutralizes, or counteracts, the change. To put it another way, a mechanism compares output with input and the system is directed to reduce the difference between the two quantities. We say that control systems of this type exhibit negative feedback. Examples of negative feedback are not limited to the regulation of internal events. For example, the intensity of human speech is adjusted to the noise level impinging upon one's own ears. Persons with deficient hearing tend to speak louder than normal.

Before considering some biological examples of internal feedback control, it is helpful to examine a simple physical system as illustrated by the thermo-statically controlled water bath. Here, the input stimulus is provided by the gain or loss of heat from the water. The resultant temperature change is detected by a piece of metal, the 'thermostat', which has a high coefficient of thermal expan-sion. The mechanical movement of the metal strip as it is warmed or cooled, opens or closes an electrical circuit which in turn operates a power supply feeding heat into the bath. The controller in this system may be equated with the thermostat. The input stimulus is the change in kinetic energy of the water molecules and the output is equated with electrical power fed into the metal coil which heats the bath.

A simple controller of this kind is responsible for an 'all or none' output. That is, the power is either full on or switched off. This is reflected in the variability in the temperature of the bath. Thus, after the heater has been switched on, there may be a time-lag before the heater begins to counteract the heat loss and the temperature of the water will continue to drop for a time. Also, after the heater has been switched off, the temperature may continue to rise through the loss of residual heat from the coil. These characteristics give rise to the phenomena of undershoot and overshoot respectively. All steady-state systems show

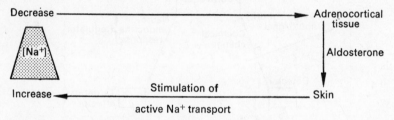

Figure 1.2. Servo-mechanism for regulation of body sodium in the frog. This feedback system is activated by a decrease in the concentration of body sodium salts. There is then an activation of the adrenocortical tissue which then secretes a hormone, aldosterone, that acts on the skin as a target, stimulating sodium transport into the body from the surrounding water.

this oscillation to a greater or lesser degree as a regular variation about a mean value. The smaller the oscillations, the more efficient is the homeostatic system.

Physiological systems differ from physical homeostatic systems mainly in the fact that all environmental changes are interpreted as chemical changes in cells and their immediate environment (Fig. 1.2). Further, the controller usually puts out a graded response which is within wide limits proportional to the magnitude of the change. This leads to a greater precision of control in that it minimizes overshoot. Another important feature of physiological homeostasis is that the initial chemical change is of minor importance against the total metabolism of the body yet it initiates a series of chemical events which culminate in a large flow of energy into the system. The entire response may be regarded as a great amplification of the initial disturbance.

Chapter 2
The Internal Environment and the Cell

General considerations

Cells are not permanent but are continuously being replaced or repaired. There is no parallel in the inanimate world of structures where repair automatically keeps pace with destruction. The best mechanical analogy of the cell is that of a moving car which is spontaneously falling apart and being put together again without an alteration in performance. Another analogy is that the organism is like a candle-flame. Just as a flame maintains its shape in a quiet atmosphere, despite the fact that wax molecules are being constantly drawn into the flame and let out as the products of burning, so the living organism maintains its form and organization despite the constant addition, degradation and excretion of its constituent molecules. Maintenance keeps pace with degradation and we say that organisms are in a steady state or in a dynamic equilibrium with their surroundings.

The cell as the fundamental unit of life may be defined in many ways, i.e. from the point of view of its structure, chemistry and reaction to stimuli. Through an assessment of the capacity of cells to respond, it is possible to account for many activities at the organ and system level.

Despite the dependence upon the composition of the extracellular phase, all cells have a greater or lesser capacity for reacting to external changes in composition and temperature in such a way as to maintain the bulk of its constituents in a constant relation, one with another. This is most clearly seen with regard to the concentration of inorganic ions and metabolites.

It is usual to stress the mechanisms for maintaining a constancy of the intracellular environment, but it is also of great importance that cells may alter their metabolism in order to maintain the key constituents at a constant level. Homeostasis does not imply an absence of change in the steady state because this may shift with time. There is no restriction on the temporal scale of homeostasis and the concept may be applied in relation to intervals ranging from milliseconds to millions of years. On the latter time scale, one is dealing with evolutionary events by which a particular organism adapts to a slowly changing environment.

Control of the steady state in cells

Maintenance of a steady state may involve a rise or fall in enzyme levels depending on the need for a greater or lesser rate of metabolism. Transient changes in chemical composition are also vital in the function of neurones, muscle and growing cells. Taking this broad view of the cellular response, it is possible to classify cellular mechanisms in the following way:

(1) Mechanisms to maintain the constancy of ions and metabolites (Movement of Water and Electrolytes);

(2) Mechanisms for the propagation of chemical change through neurones (The Nerve Impulse);

(3) Mechanisms to control enzyme activity (Control of Enzymes);

(4) Mechanisms to control the size and numbers of cells (Growth and Cell Division);

(5) Mechanisms for controlling cell shape (Muscular Contraction and Movement).

Each of these topics will now be considered in detail.

Movement of water and electrolytes

One of the characteristics of the body fluids of all types of multicellular organisms is that they contain sodium and potassium as the two major inorganic constituents. Another generalization may be made that sodium is a characteristic component of the extracellular fluids, whilst potassium is mainly confined within the cells. From studies on the composition of the extracellular fluids of a wide range of metazoans, it appears that the concentration of K^+ lies either in the range 4 to 6 mequiv/l, or between 10 and 16 mequiv/l. The lower values are found in organisms that inhabit fresh water and land, whilst the higher values are found in marine forms. The sodium concentration in the extracellular fluids is more variable than that of potassium, and organisms can be divided into three groups: those which have Na^+ concentrations of approximately 40, 150 and 450 mequiv/l. These divisions roughly correspond to organisms living in fresh water, fresh water and land, and sea water, respectively. This generalization comes mainly from work on the invertebrates, but departures from the rule are found in the vertebrates which live in a marine environment, where the sodium content of the extracellular fluids resembles that of their freshwater or terrestrial ancestors. In all cases, however, the extracellular fluids have a higher concentration of sodium than do the fluids of the cells. Conversely, the cell fluids always have a higher concentration of potassium than do the extracellular fluids. This may be expressed as the rule of differential distribution of ions, and is a constant feature of organisms in their normal environment.

If the differences in composition between the intracellular and the extracellular fluids are compared with compartmented non-living systems, a basic difference can be found that points to a unique feature of the cell membrane that divides the two solutions. In a non-living system, when two solutions that differ in composition are separated by a partition through which the dissolved substances pass, that is, the partition or boundary membrane is permeable to these substances, the two solutions will equilibrate by the process of diffusion.

Diffusion is the movement of molecules resulting from their intrinsic kinetic energy. These effects of molecular movement may be observed in a solution by adding particles to it that are just visible with the light microscope, for example, the carbon particles in ink. Because bombardment of the carbon particles by the molecules of the solution is not equal in all directions, the particles gradually move about at random. This phenomenon is termed Brownian motion.

If an aqueous solution of a substance A is separated from an aqueous solution of substance B by a membrane that is permeable to both A and B, then initially there will be a high chance of A and B passing through the membrane out of their initial compartments and a low chance that they will pass back again. Thus, there will be a net movement of A in one direction, and a net movement of B in the other direction. This is another way of saying that the chances of A and B moving out of their original compartments are proportional to their concentrations in those compartments. Gradually, as their concentrations increase in the second compartment, there will be an increasing chance that random movements will result in these molecules returning to their original compartments. Eventually, when the concentration of A and B is the same in compartments 1 and 2, the chance of movement of A in each direction will be the same and there will be no net change in concentration, although molecules will be continually passing back and forth between the two compartments. At this point, we say that the two solutions are in equilibrium. For any two solutions of different composition separated by a permeable membrane, a mixing of the two solutions will occur by movement of substances from a high concentration to a low concentration, until the composition of both solutions is the same. In this phenomenon of diffusion, substances are said to move down their concentration gradients.

Osmotic pressure

If the membrane does not allow one of the solutes to pass through it is termed a semi-permeable membrane. Consider a situation where the total pressure is initially the same on each side of the membrane; an aqueous solution of a solute A is separated from pure water by a membrane which allows water molecules to pass through it. More water molecules bombard the membrane per unit time on the pure water side; the water on the solution side may be regarded as being 'diluted' by the solute. Therefore, more water molecules cross into the solution than move in the opposite direction, giving a net flow into the solution.

The system can only come into equilibrium when the pressure of water, due to diffusion and hydrostatic pressure, is the same in both compartments. When this equilibrium is attained, the difference in total pressure on both sides of the membrane is termed the osmotic pressure of the solution and is a measure of the pressure exerted by the given concentration of solute.

At low concentrations of solute, the osmotic pressure is the same as the pressure exerted by a perfect gas at the same concentration and temperature.

$$\text{Osmotic pressure (dynes/cm}^2) = R.T.c.$$

$R = $ Gas constant (ergs/degree/mole)
$T = $ Absolute temperature
$c = $ Solute concentration (moles/cm^3)

The total osmotic pressure for a solution containing a number of solutes is the sum of the contributions made by each particle type, just as pressure of mixed gases is the sum of their partial pressures. When calculating the osmotic pressure of mixed solutions, it is necessary to work out the number of different species, both undissociated salt and its ions, using the appropriate dissociation constant. It is generally accepted that the cell contents of multicellular organisms are at the same osmotic pressure (isosmotic) as the extracellular fluid. Differences in osmotic pressure are found at the boundary membranes at the body surface, for example, the gill of fish or the intestinal epithelium, of aquatic organisms and the body fluids may have a lower (hyposmotic) or higher (hyperosmotic) osmotic pressure than the external solutions. Thus, water leaves or enters the body and these osmotic losses or gains must be counterbalanced by special mechanisms.

Active transport

If the cell membrane is permeable to both Na^+ and K^+, one would expect mixing to occur by diffusion until there were equal concentrations of Na^+ and K^+ in both compartments. In fact, an unequal salt distribution is maintained and this suggests that these two ions cannot pass through the membrane; that is, it is impermeable to Na^+ and K^+. This possibility can be tested experimentally.

Individual isolated muscles from higher animals are found to be composed predominantly of cells with little extracellular material and so are useful in carrying out test-tube investigations into the mechanisms of ionic regulation. To test the possibility that intracellular K^+ is able to move down its diffusion gradient out of the cell, the diffusion gradient can be exaggerated by placing an intact muscle in a solution for the most part resembling plasma, but containing no K^+. In this artificial medium, it is found that over a period of several hours, K^+ gradually leaves the muscle and appears in the medium. At the same time as the K^+ is lost, the tissue takes up an equivalent amount of Na^+ from the external solution. Thus, in this one experiment, it is shown that the cell membrane is permeable to both ions. The observation that the number of sodium ions that enter the muscle is equal to the number of potassium ions lost, indicates that a negatively charged ion remains behind when the positively charged K^+ leaves the muscle; Na^+ enters the cell attracted to this indiffusible anion.

However, it is possible that the conclusions drawn from the last experiment may not be valid for the intact animal, because the muscle was placed in an environment that it would never encounter in life. A second technique may be used to overcome the limitation imposed by the use of these 'test-tube' conditions. Radioactive isotopes of both sodium and potassium can be prepared and used as markers of the movement of these ions in the body. Immediately after the intravenous injection of small quantities of highly radioactive sodium or potassium into higher vertebrates, most of the isotope appears in the blood. Thereafter, the concentration in the blood decreases and the concentration in the cells rises. This change occurs without any measurable change in the concentration of the total ions in either fluid compartment. Eventually, an equilibrium point is reached after which the concentration of isotope in both blood and cells decreases as the radioactive ions are excreted in the urine. It is important in this kind of experiment that the quantity of labelled ions should be very small in comparison with the total quantity of ions in the body. Only in this way can it be ensured that the results are not affected by abnormal concentration gradients being set up.

Isotope experiments of this type show that both Na^+ and K^+ readily cross the cell membrane in both directions. Thus, faced with a freely permeable membrane, how are the gradients for Na^+ and K^+ maintained? The most likely answer is that as sodium ions enter the cell down the diffusion gradient, these ions are pushed out again to maintain a constant level in the cell. For K^+, we may postulate a similar mechanism to replace the potassium ions that leave the cell down their diffusion gradient. The phenomenon of movement of ions against the direction of the diffusion gradient is termed active transport. It may be likened to a process that tends to concentrate ions and so is akin to the physical phenomenon of evaporation and compression; these processes require energy and in the same way, active transport is an energy-requiring process. When the movements of ions against diffusion or concentration gradients are discussed, the cellular mechanism is likened to a pump; that is, intracellular Na^+ is pumped out of the cell and extracellular K^+ is pumped in. It is likely that Na^+ and K^+ pumps are located in the cell membrane.

Energy and active transport

Cells may be studied in isolation from the body in the form of thin slices of tissues or as blood cells isolated from the plasma and suspended in an inorganic medium.

The normal concentration of cell K^+ in such cells may be lowered by immersing them for a time in a K^+-free medium. On returning these K^+ depleted cells to a solution containing the normal amounts of Na^+ and K^+ found in blood plasma, the cells begin to pump out the accumulated Na^+ and regain K^+, so in this way it is possible to measure active transport as a *net* movement of ions. Using this kind of cellular system, it has been shown that the Na^+ pump utilizes as the direct energy source the compound adenosinetriphosphate (ATP), which is formed by normal metabolic reactions. In red blood cells, for example, on average, between 1 to 2 sodium ions are transported per molecule of ATP utilized.

Special developments of the sodium pump

The Na^+ pump appears to be basic to all cells as part of the mechanism whereby the cell maintains a constant intracellular concentration of Na^+ and K^+. However, modifications of the ion transport system occur in several cell types as an important part of their specialized functions. The modifications considered below are of two kinds. First, mechanisms for regulating the concentration of Na^+ in the extracellular fluid. These mechanisms all require the polarization of the transport process for unidirectional transport and are found in cells at the boundary between body and environment. That is, instead of functioning to maintain a constant ratio of intracellular to extracellular Na^+, as in most cells of the body, the pump carries out the net transport of Na^+ through the cells, into or out of the body. According to the direction of the transport, these systems may be divided up as follows:

Inward transport	e.g. Frog skin
	Plant roots
Inward or outward transport	e.g. Kidney in vertebrates
	Gills in fish and crustacea
Outward transport	e.g. Salt gland in birds and reptiles
	Rectal gland in cartilaginous fish

The second important adaptation of the Na^+ pump occurs in the nerve axons and muscles of animals. Here Na^+ transport plays a central role in the transmission of the nerve impulses and the initiation of the contractile process in muscle. Examples of these two kinds of adaptation will be considered in detail below.

The frog skin

About the middle of the nineteenth century it was observed that skin taken from a frog and stretched as a partition between two compartments containing NaCl solution at equal concentrations, maintained an electrical potential difference between its inner and outer surface. The potential difference was measured by placing silver wires in each compartment and connecting them together through a voltmeter. The compartment corresponding to the inner surface of the skin was positive to the compartment in contact with the outer surface. Voltages generated by skin are very small and are expressed in millivolts (1 mV = 1/1000 V). Thus, from this early work, the isolated skin was likened to a battery in that a small but measurable current could be drawn from it. Later, it was found that to demonstrate the potential difference, it was essential that the external compartment contained NaCl; the internal compartment could contain pure water. This indicated that the current drawn from the inside of the skin was due to the movement of positively charged sodium ions from the outer compartment. Later still, it was found that isolated skin carried out the continuous transport of NaCl from the outer to the inner surface. Also, transport took place even if conditions were arranged so that the concentration of NaCl in the inner compartment was much higher than that outside. Thus, skin cells appeared to contain an active transport system which could pump sodium ions, with chloride ions following passively. A slight lag between the passage of the positively charged sodium ions and the negatively charged chloride ions would account for the slight excess of positive charges inside the skin. By connecting up the two sides of the skin with a conducting wire, the excess of chloride ions on the outside of the skin give up their electrons and form silver chloride, the electrons passing through the wire to the inner solution where they combine with hydrogen ions of water to form hydrogen atoms. The sodium ions are neutralized by the remaining excess hydroxyls.

By experiment, it is possible to establish a relationship between the number of ions transported in any system, living or non-living, and the current that can be drawn from the system. For a chemical reaction of the type that produces current in a battery, Faraday established that the transport of 1 g equivalent of any ion is associated with a definite quantity of electricity called a Faraday (F). If the current is measured in amps then the smallest standard quantity of electricity is the coulomb (1 F = 96,500 coulombs). Coulombs are obtained by multiplying the current in amps by the time in seconds during which this current is drawn from the system (1 coulomb is equivalent to 1/96,500th of a gram equivalent). In frog skin experiments, the current that can be drawn from the skin lies between 10 and 100 milli-coulombs.

The maximum current obtained from a piece of skin is measured practically by connecting a battery to the skin so that the current produced by the battery opposes that normally produced by the skin (Fig. 2.1). The current applied from the external circuit, A, is adjusted until there is no drop in voltage across the skin, V, which means that electrons are being supplied from the battery to neutralize the transported sodium ions. At this point, the current in the external circuit equals the current produced by the skin, and it is said to be in 'short circuit'. It is of interest to compare the short-circuit current with the number of sodium ions transported by the skin at the same time that the current is measured. As the net sodium movement is quite slow, chemical analysis is not sufficiently sensitive to determine the rate of transport and it is necessary to use a radioactive isotope of sodium as a label. When skin is set up so that it resembles the condition in the animal, that is with a high concentration of Na^+ on the inside and a low concentration of Na^+ on the outside, Na^+ moves passively through the skin down the diffusion gradient from inside to outside. In order to determine the net transport of Na^+ inwards, it is necessary to measure the inward (active) and outward (passive) movement of Na^+ simultaneously. This is achieved by using two different isotopes of sodium that can be determined by separate methods and adding one to the inner chamber and the other to the outer chamber. Only net Na^+ movement would be expected to produce a current, and the

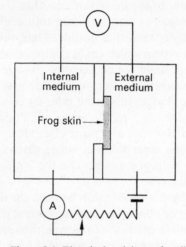

Figure 2.1. Electrical activity and sodium transport by frog skin.

results of this kind of experiment show that the current flowing at any time is exactly equal to the number of sodium ions that arise as a balance between active transport and back diffusion.

The biological significance of Na^+ transport in the skin of amphibia is that the frog in pond water loses NaCl from the body fluids by outward diffusion through the skin, and by excretion in the urine. The Na^+ pump in the cells of the skin enables the animal to offset these losses by taking in NaCl dissolved in pond water. The feedback system is detailed in Fig. 1.2. The stimulus to the receptor is a drop in the Na^+ concentration of body fluids through the loss of Na^+ through the skin (passive) and kidney (filtration of plasma). The controller is a group of hormone-producing cells, the adrenocortical tissue, and the output is the release of the hormone aldosterone from these cells. Aldosterone makes more energy available to the Na^+ pumps in the skin (the regulator) and this results in an increased net uptake of sodium through the skin.

Urine is stored in the bladder of amphibians and the bladder cells are also able to transport urinary sodium actively back into the body. This ion transport process, like that in skin, is also sensitive to aldosterone.

In all transport processes, the transport of a cation is associated either with the movement of an equal number of anions (sometimes also an active process) in the same direction or the movement of an equal number of other cations in the opposite direction.

In general, it may be said that hormones form an essential link between controller and regulator (Fig. 1.2). The other means by which animals co-ordinate responses to their environment is through the nervous system. Indeed, if the hormones are regarded as chemical messengers, nerves may be regarded as special structures which enable a chemical change to be rapidly transmitted to specific organs for appropriate responses. The essential chemical nature of the nerve impulse will now be discussed because the underlying basic mechanism is that of active Na^+ transport.

The nerve impulse

Frog skin may be used as an example to demonstrate how ion transport processes may give rise to electrical activity in cellular systems. In this case, the potential difference is measured across a sheet of tissue composed of several layers of cells. Electrical activity is actually a feature of all cells and may be measured by inserting an electrode into the cell and putting a second electrode in the extra-cellular fluid. The potential difference between the two electrodes is a function of the cell membrane: the intracellular environment being slightly negative to the extracellular fluid. This phenomenon would be expected if there were slightly less positively charged ions in the cell compared with negative ones.

Let us examine a model system of the ion distribution across the cell membrane (Fig. 2.2). Two compartments are imagined, 1 and 2, containing equal volumes of KCl solution. Compartment 1 also contains the potassium salt of an acid, A. All of these compounds are fully dissociated and we start the experiment in the situation shown in Fig. 2.2, where each symbol represents one equivalent of the ion. An important assumption is made that the membrane separating the two solutions is permeable to K^+ and Cl^-, but not to A^-. When a membrane allows the differential movement of ions we say it is semi-permeable.

At the start of the experiment, the concentration of K^+ in Compartment 1 is higher than the K^+ concentration in Compartment 2 (2:1). Thus, there is a diffusion gradient for K^+ loss from the first compartment. Potassium ions will therefore move out and chloride ions will tend to follow them. However, as soon as chloride ions enter Compartment 2, there will be a diffusion gradient for the loss of Cl^- from this compartment. Actually, the rate of K^+ movement will be hindered by the presence of A^- in Compartment 1, which since it cannot move through the membrane, will hold back potassium ions by electrostatic attraction. Eventually, a state of equilibrium will be set up in which the rate of K^+ loss from

Compartment 1 by diffusion is balanced by the electrostatic attraction to the chloride and acid ions in Compartment 1. At the equilibrium point, the concentration of K^+ will be higher in 1 than 2; conversely, the concentration of Cl^- will be higher in 2 than in 1 and there will be a slight excess of unbalanced negative charges in Compartment 1 due to the presence of A^- which cannot pass through the membrane. This indiffusible anion is responsible for the potential difference. In the body the phenomenon of the cell potential is caused by the presence of negatively charged indiffusible cell protein and is termed the Donnan Effect. For any ion that has an uneven distribution across a membrane, it is

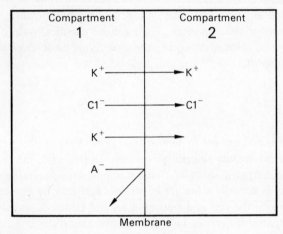

Figure 2.2. Model representing differential distribution of potassium salts across the cell membrane and direction of diffusion gradients.

possible to calculate the membrane potential by means of an equation which takes into consideration the concentration ratio of each diffusible ion across the membrane.

Membrane potentials of most cells in the multicellular organism are usually constant at about -70 mV. However, if electrodes are arranged across the membrane of a nerve cell, a periodic drop in the membrane potential may be observed. The oscillation lasts less than a second and then there is a return of the potential to normal (Fig. 2.3). A rapidly reversible variation of this kind is called an action potential and is associated with the passage of a nerve impulse along a nerve cell. Sometimes the impulse results in the abolition of the membrane potential, when we say that the nerve is depolarized. On other occasions the potential is reversed so that the inside becomes positive relative to the outside. If the long process of the nerve (the axon) remains connected to the muscle which it normally innervates, the action potential may be traced as it passes along the nerve and into the muscle fibres. When the wave of depolarization reaches the muscle, the muscle contracts.

Axons in higher vertebrates are generally too small for experimental purposes (between 0·5 and 5·0 μm in diameter) and most of the work has been carried out on the much larger 'giant axon' of the squid. Apart from their size, the giant axons are also of great value for experiments in that they can be taken from the body and still maintain their conducting properties when immersed in sea water for a very long period.

By means of electrical measurements after manipulations of the external and internal environment of isolated squid axons, it has been possible to establish the

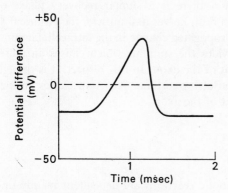

Figure 2.3. Action potential in nerve.

sequence of events at a particular point on the axon during the passage of the impulse.

The axon membrane, like the outer membranes of other cells, is characterized by a Na^+ pump which maintains steady-state concentration gradients of K^+ and Na^+ between the intra- and extracellular fluids. Normally, the rate of Na^+ entry is quite low compared with that of K^+ (only about one tenth as fast). When the impulse reaches a particular region of the axon, there is first a very large increase in the permeability of the membrane to Na^+. The Na^+ pump cannot cope with the greatly increased inflow of sodium ions and there is a fall in the membrane potential as these ions neutralize the negative charges on the intracellular protein. The gradient for Na^+ entry may be so large that the axon ends up with an excess of sodium ions and becomes positively charged with respect to the outside. This phase of high Na^+ permeability is short-lived and is followed by a return to the normal low state of permeability. Under these conditions, the axon now contains too many positive ions and moves to a new state of equilibrium through the loss of potassium ions equivalent to the sodium ions that entered. This phase of K efflux corresponds with the restoration of the normal membrane potential. The whole process involving Na^+/K^+ exchange lasts about 1 millisecond. During the passage of each impulse along the axon, the nerve loses about a millionth of its total K^+ and gains an equal amount of Na^+. This small increase in the concentration of sodium is the basic chemical change which is transmitted along the axon.

So far, we have considered changes in permeability that do not involve energy consumption. However, in order to restore the lost K^+ the axon must take up ions against a concentration gradient. Also, the additional intracellular Na^+ gained during the passage of the action potential must be extruded. It is during the next phase, the recovery phase, that the Na^+ pump brings about a net exchange of intracellular Na^+ for K^+, utilizing ATP formed in the aerobic reactions of electron transport.

A similar increase in Na^+ permeability of the muscle fibres appears to initiate muscular contraction and there is a similar recovery phase of Na^+ extrusion in exchange for K^+. In both nerves and muscle, the electrical activity is simply a manifestation of a propagated change in the intracellular concentrations of Na^+ and K^+ that provides the stimulus which causes an increase in permeability of the next segment of the axon. In this respect, it is thought that it is the rise in the concentration of intracellular Na^+ that causes an increased permeability of the next segment of the axon.

The control of enzymes

The direction and rate of metabolic reactions are dependent mainly upon the relative concentration of enzyme and substrate molecules. Thus, control may be exerted in two ways: by changes in the concentration of the substrates and products of the enzyme, or by changes in the concentration and catalytic activity of the enzymes. The metabolism of glucose by cell-free extracts, for example, may be controlled by varying the concentration of the major reactants; glucose, phosphate ions, ATP and nicotinamide adenine dinucleotide (NAD) (Fig. 2.4).

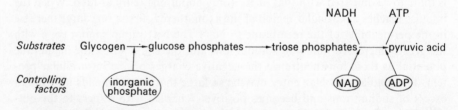

Figure 2.4. Factors controlling the metabolism of glucose.

Also, the rate of reaction will be decreased if the cell-free extract is diluted before addition of the reactants, showing the inhibitory effect of lowering the enzyme concentration. In the cell, metabolic reactions are more closely knit together and the rate of removal of ATP to give adenosine diphosphate (ADP) by any energy-requiring reactions will, by changing the concentration of ADP as a phosphate acceptor in the glycolytic pathway, control the rate of glucose utilization. In this way, energy production keeps pace with energy utilization.

In general, enzymes are more active in cell-free preparations than they are in the cell. The reason for this is that enzymes are held in various intracellular structures so that enzyme and substrate do not mix readily. For example, the oxidative enzymes of the citric acid cycle are confined to particles called mitochondria, whilst their major supply of substrate, which comes from glycolysis, is controlled by extramitochondrial enzymes. Also, the membrane of the mitochondria is not freely permeable to substrates of the citric acid cycle. It is those compounds, such as ATP, which are present at a limiting concentration that offer the best possibility for the fine and rapid control of metabolism.

With regard to effects on enzymes, quick-acting activators of metabolism often work by altering the structure of an enzyme to make it more or less efficient as a catalyst (allosteric effects). On the other hand, changes in enzyme concentration or membrane structure (permeability) often take several hours or even days to become effective.

Many metabolites are capable of inhibiting enzymes, particularly if they are tightly bound to the enzyme. If such a metabolite is the product of the enzyme, the enzyme becomes less active as the reaction proceeds and eventually the reaction may cease altogether. The enzyme may be activated when the product is removed. In the cell, this takes place naturally through the activity of another enzyme which uses the inhibitor as a substrate. This form of control is common in enzymes which form a chain, breaking down a substrate into necessarily smaller units. Sometimes, one of the terminal products of the enzyme sequence is an inhibitor of one of the enzymes responsible for an early step. This mechanism, called feedback control inhibition, is of great importance in cellular metabolism.

As an example, we may take the case of the bacterium *Escherichia coli* making the amino acid, histidine. This process requires eight different enzymes working in sequence. If excess histidine is added to the culture, the bacterium stops making histidine because the amino acid inhibits the first enzyme in the biosynthetic pathway. Many of the succeeding steps require energy and it is clearly economical to stop the reaction at the first step if histidine is plentiful.

Histidine is made by *E. coli* in order to satisfy part of a requirement for amino acids which may be assembled into proteins. Some of these proteins will be enzymes and their synthesis may also be regulated by the nutrients in the environment. For example, certain strains of *E. coli* grown on glucose and ammonia as the only source for assembling the entire range of compounds of carbon and nitrogen, cannot make immediate use of other sugars as a source of carbon.

The disaccharide lactose cannot be used because the bacterium does not possess the enzyme β-galactosidase which breaks lactose into glucose and galactose. However, after a time in the presence of lactose, cells which have been grown only on glucose can make use of lactose as the sole source of carbon compounds. During the lag period before lactose can be utilized, the enzyme β-galactoside is formed which is a new and specific protein. Such an enzyme is termed an inducible or adaptive enzyme, in contrast to the constitutive enzymes which are always present. The substrate, lactose in this instance, which initiates the synthesis of the inducible enzyme, is called an inducer. Inducers are usually specific for a particular enzyme. Although it is not always the case that an inducer is a metabolite of the induced enzyme they usually bear close structural relationships with the substrate of the enzyme.

Through a slight change in a bacterial genotype by, for example, irradiation, it is possible to change an inducible enzyme into a constitutive one. This gives rise to the hypothesis that there are two kinds of genes controlling enzyme synthesis. One type is termed a structural gene, which is thought of as controlling the basic steps in the synthesis of the enzyme. The other kind is termed a regulating gene; these are concerned with activating and inactivating the structural genes. The hypothesis also states that regulatory genes produce substances known as repressors which are the immediate cause of inhibition of structural genes. Thus, to complete the theory, an inducer brings about the synthesis of a specific enzyme by combining, either with the regulatory gene to prevent the formation of the repressor, or with the repressor itself to render it inactive. Either of these events is envisaged as allowing protein synthesis to occur under the control of a structural gene (Fig. 2.5).

The fact that a cell may contain a particular enzyme does not guarantee that it can utilize the substrate of that enzyme if this is present in the extracellular environment. Cells are often unable to use substrates because the compounds cannot pass the cell membrane. The process of induction is probably very important in the exercise of selectivity at the cell boundary. For example, many substrates enter bacteria by the operation of active transport systems termed permeases. These systems respond to environmental and genetic influences in much the same way as do inducible enzymes. Thus, permeases provide another group of regulatory mechanisms for cellular metabolism.

The three modes of metabolic control by feedback inhibition, repression and induction are clearly seen to be of importance in the day-to-day life of bacteria, but are also found to be a characteristic of all organisms. The phenomenon of induction would be advantageous at any stage in evolution in that enzyme synthesis, which is expensive in terms of energy, would be geared to the need for the enzymes. This is most obvious when we discern the process of induction as a specific response to the external environment, but it is probably also of great importance in the intracellular regulation of enzyme levels to ensure the integration of the many biochemical pathways.

Growth and cell division

In general, when a cell grows to twice its original mass or volume, it divides into two and the two daughter cells repeat this cycle. This doubling of size between 'birth' and division suggests that there is a control mechanism which 'measures'

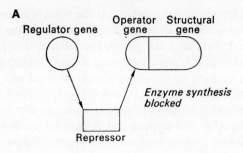

A

Regulator gene   Operator   Structural
               gene   gene

*Enzyme synthesis
blocked*

Repressor

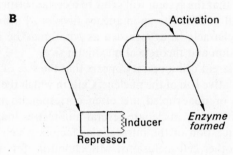

B

Activation

Inducer

*Enzyme
formed*

Repressor

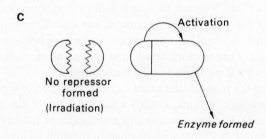

C

Activation

No repressor
formed

(Irradiation)

Enzyme formed

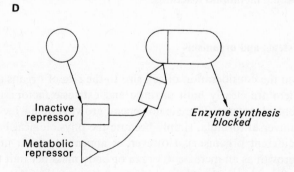

D

Inactive
repressor

Metabolic
repressor

*Enzyme synthesis
blocked*

Figure 2.5. Three types of gene regulation of enzyme synthesis (B–D).

the size of a cell. One of the factors limiting cell size is the relative surface area because the rate of internal processes is dependent upon the exchange of substances at the cell surface and then, as a cell grows, the relative area per unit mass decreases. In this connection, it is possible from a simple consideration of the physical prerequisites of division to construct a mathematical cell model, consisting of a droplet where import and export, together with anabolism and catabolism of materials take place. Within such a system, concentration gradients of substances entering and leaving will appear and it may be predicted that these gradients will lead to forces tending to disrupt the system and counteract division. It can be shown also that the system will grow to a certain critical value where metabolic forces prevail and lead to spontaneous division. From such a droplet system a number of characteristics regarded as 'vital' may be derived, such as growth, periodic division and theoretical maximum size.

From a comparison of different cell types, it appears that the size of a cell is dependent mainly upon the relative size of the nucleus. Cells in which the nuclear substance has been doubled or quadrupled are often correspondingly large. Moreover, protozoan cells with many nuclei are several millimetres long.

In addition, there is the question of the intracellular factors which control the number and size of the other cell inclusions. Mitochondria, for instance, grow and divide. Also, chloroplasts in lower plants have been observed to multiply by fission, each of which grows to a well-defined maximum size. The average number of both of these organelles is regulated intracellularly in relation to need. In this respect, both chloroplasts and mitochondria have been shown to contain the genetic material of the nucleus, DNA, and this is true of other bodies which also divide, such as basal granules of cilia and flagella.

The general idea is that the nucleus and other cell particles receive signals or stimuli from the cytoplasm and, in turn, modify their influence of the growth process in the rest of the cell. The exact nature of these signals is unknown, but they are likely to be chemical in nature and to operate through feedback processes to modify specific metabolic reactions.

Growth in organ systems and organisms

When we move from the consideration of cell size to the size of organs and the entire organism, there are clearly both intrinsic and extrinsic factors at work which operate as control systems. There is no general growth curve which could be expressed in a universal formula, simply because the physiological basis for growth differs in different organisms. However, it appears to be a universal characteristic that growth as an increase in organ or body mass per unit time, is not unlimited. As a general rule, there is a rapid increase in mass which gradually slows down until the organism reaches a stage where it is adult. The limitation of growth is not, in principle, due to a decline in the growth potency of the component cells or tissues, but rather it is regulated by factors acting within the organism. This is evident because cells which have stopped growing and multiplying in the adult organism may resume growth and multiplication if the internal balance is altered to provoke the phenomena of regeneration, compensatory hyperplasia or growth in tissue culture.

In insects, the individual cells of tissues and organs (with the major exception of the central nervous system) are in contact with their neighbours in only two dimensions, since epithelial sheets and cylinders are used to obtain complexity rather than the three dimensional masses of cells utilized by most other metazoa. Thus the varieties of body form in insects are the result of the activities of a single layer of epidermal cells, expressed through the secretion and modification of the cuticular exoskeleton. Moreover, this sheet of cells determines the form and pattern characteristic of successive instars, culminating in the specific form of the adult body.

It is obvious that insect epidermal cells have an outside, on which the cuticle is secreted, and an inside, from which the precursors of cuticle formation are extracted from the blood. What is less clear is the ultrastructural basis for this organization of the cell. Further, transplantation of pieces of epidermis, sometimes with rotation of the grafts, has revealed that the insect epidermal cell has an antero-posterior orientation and, in addition, is organized relative to its position in a transverse line of cells. Little is known of the structural basis for this orientation, except that it results from the action of polarized gradients and fields, perhaps related to the presence of septate desmosomes which provide channels for intercommunication between the cells. The final result of these interactions is that the position and functions of individual cells is determined both in the segments and in the appendages, and thus in the body overall. The whole epidermal sheet can thereby be considered as a unit, with development and change in one part influencing similar processes elsewhere. The individual potentialities of a single cell are therefore conditioned by the properties which groups of cells superimpose upon themselves. The specific orientations of epidermal cells are lost—sometimes only temporarily—when they divide and migrate to heal wounds.

The developmental changes which take place in successive instars to achieve the adult body form are initiated by hormones, acting in some way upon the genetic constitution of the epidermal cells. But the reaction of an individual cell to the presence of such hormones is still dependent upon its position in the body and the overall response of its neighbours. For example, the number of divisions which an epidermal cell in the thorax will undergo at a moult may be greatly in excess of that of an abdominal cell. In essentially the same way, although responding more subtly to local influences, differences in bristle pattern and number, density of dermal glands, pigmentation, and so on, can arise in successive instars not only because of the fluctuating hormonal status of the instars, but also because the changes occur in the context of the cellular environment.

The existence of polarized gradients and fields in vertebrate embryogenesis is well established; their operation during insect metamorphosis may well be an extension of processes begun in the egg. They do serve, however, to emphasize the importance of cellular interactions in the metazoan body, which may be quite independent of well-recognized communication media such as the blood and nervous systems.

Notwithstanding its detailed complexity, the growth process in the organism as a whole can be defined in relatively simple quantitative expressions and this has led to the formulation of several theories on the control of growth. One of the more biochemically orientated models is that of Drs. Weiss and Kavanau, which has as its central idea that each cell produces inhibitors which prevent the growth and division of the cells that release them into the extracellular fluid. Hence, there is a negative feedback system where growth leads to growth inhibition and the attainment of a terminal size is an expression of a steady state, controlled partly through self-reproducing templates (the cells) and freely diffusible antitemplates (growth inhibitors). There is some experimental evidence that inhibitors of this nature (termed 'chalones') are an important factor in regulating organ size, particularly in the case of mammalian liver.

The crucial observation involves the experimental removal of part of a liver lobe. Over a period of a fortnight the total mass of the remaining liver gradually increases and becomes stabilized at the weight that it was before the operation. More detailed experiments involving the dilution and concentration of blood plasma have indicated that liver growth is inhibited by factors produced by the liver, i.e. when the quantity of circulating inhibitor is reduced by taking out part of the liver tissue or by diluting the plasma, the liver begins to grow.

In micro-organisms, alterations in the external environment play an important direct role in regulating growth and development. On the other hand, in a higher animal or plant, growth and development are regulated by an orderly succession of different internal environments which are, in turn, governed by heredity. There is a succession of events in development produced through the action of complex feedback mechanisms which, as well as involving regulation of gene action, also involves the activity of various growth-promoting hormones.

Muscular contraction and movement

Many cell types, whether or not they are capable of movement, exhibit a streaming or flow of their contents. Both the extent of streaming and the extent and direction of movement are affected by environmental factors. Flow occurs because the contents of cells have much in common with the physical state described as a liquid crystal or paracrystalline state. All paracrystalline substances have elongated molecules or groups of protein molecules. These rod-like, submicroscopic particles are termed micellae and are able to line up along one axis and slide freely over each other in the direction of the plane of alignment. The importance of the paracrystalline state is that it has the advantages of fluidity and diffusibility common to liquids but, most important, has the possibility of leading to the spatial organization of the cell contents in one, two or three dimensions.

Streaming movements in cells carry along the submicroscopic organelles such as mitochondria and chloroplasts. It is but a short step from cyclosis, the continuous flow around the periphery of the cell, to movement of the whole cell. Movement by a change in form, amoeboid movement, occurs by the continuous build-up of material at the 'front' end whilst, at the same time, the 'hind' end is shortening as material is withdrawn into the interior. Amoeboid movement is analogous to the progression of a caterpillar tractor where treads are lifted up from the rear and placed in front on a continuous belt. Each tread remains stationary whilst in contact with the ground in a similar way to that in amoeboid movement, each portion of the cell membrane in contact with the underlying surface remains stationary. Cells change direction by a cessation of flow followed by the re-establishment of flow in a different direction.

Various explanations and models have been set up to explain amoeboid movement, but none is wholly satisfactory. It is clear, however, that the energy is provided by metabolic reactions.

With regard to the present discussion, the point at issue is the stimulus which evokes cell movement. The operation of this stimulus may be seen in the healing of wounds, particularly in insects. If the epidermis is cut, the injured cells die and some product of the autolysis of these cells leads to the activation of the surrounding cells over a wide zone, up to 800 μm radius, around the point of injury. These activated cells are attracted and migrate to the margin of the wound, creating a sparse zone at the periphery. Cell movement following injury may be looked upon as a homeostatic reaction to make good the loss of continuity of the epidermal sheet of cells. In the sparse zone, mitoses appear about five days after the injury; subsequent division and increase in size of the cells restores the normal cell density. Here we have a homeostatic response which is made up of two processes: cell migration and cell division. The homeostatic migration is brought to an end by the restoration of continuity; mitosis is brought to an end by the restoration of normal cell density.

Apart from the bulk flow of cytoplasm as a reaction to stimuli, movement in response to the environment is achieved in multicellular organisms by localized contractions of groups of muscle cells acting in unison. Also, micro-organisms and many multicellular organisms make use of special cell processes capable of directed movement, termed flagella and cilia. The same basic chemical response is thought to underlie all of these systems.

Contractibility of cells, which is clearly responsible for mechanical movement, is not fully understood, but it is known that in the process of contraction, ATP is broken down to ADP. This intrinsic ATP-utilizing mechanism may be demonstrated in glycerol-extracted muscles and flagellated organisms when ATP is added to them. Extracted muscles, flagella and cilia beat rhythmically despite the fact that most of the soluble cell contents have been removed.

When a muscle contracts, it shortens and increases in thickness. Several hypotheses have been put forward to explain this phenomenon, but the one which has most support at the moment comes from studies of the ultrastructure of skeletal muscle. Basically, it supposes that a muscle shortens by a process in which two sets of straight fibres interdigitate like the coming together of the fingers of two hands. There are two kinds of fibres composed largely of two separate insoluble proteins, termed actin and myosin. The chemical mechanism proposes that each thin actin fibre slides along a thick myosin fibre, possibly by the alternate making and breaking of bonds between the two proteins. Further, it is thought that movement of each fibre relative to the other is initiated by a change in ionic composition of the muscle cell after the nerve action potential is transmitted to the muscle.

Part II
Adaptations at the Interface between Organism and Environment

Chapter 3
The Epidermis

General

In all metazoa, the outer layer of body cells derived from the embryonic ecto-derm forms a boundary between the individual and its external environment. This epidermis must originally have been the site of gaseous exchange in respira-tion, the layer across which the waste products of metabolism diffused, and also, as a result of the development of cilia, the means by which the organism moved in its fluid environment. Moreover, the epidermal layer, in direct contact with the environment, must have been used to appreciate external changes so that sense organs, and early on, a nervous system which later invaginated, were formed from this layer.

Many of the original functions of the epidermis are retained to this day in some animal groups. Thus the entire skin of an earthworm functions as a res-piratory organ, although in the polychaetes specialized blood and coelomic gills are developed so that gaseous exchange is restricted to particular areas of the epidermis. In crustaceans, similarly, the whole body surface serves for respira-tion in all larvae, and also in adult branchiopods, ostracods, free-living copepods, and many cirripedes; in the Branchiura Thermosbaenacea, mysids and tanaids, gaseous exchange takes place mainly at the surface of the carapace, whereas epidermal gills are developed in other groups. In the tracheate arthropods, the tracheae are invaginations of the epidermis.

Ctenophores, some turbellarians and nemertines, and rotifers retain the power of ciliary locomotion. But many animals with a ciliated epidermis use their cilia not for movement through water but to draw water towards them—the same *relative* purpose. Such mechanisms are found in many coelenterates, sedentary polychaetes, molluscs, crinoids, ascidians, *Amphioxus* and the ammo-coete larvae of lampreys.

The excretory function of the epidermis in modern animals is exemplified best by the ectodermal invaginations forming the nephridia in polychaetes. However, in this group there are various degrees of fusion between nephridia and the mesodermal coelomoducts—forming nephromixia—and in many anne-lid species as in some arthropods, the coelomoducts have to a large extent taken over the excretory function. Similarly, the ectodermal sense organs frequently have important mesodermal components in many animals, particularly the vertebrates.

In animals with increasing complexity of organization, where homeostatic control of the internal environment becomes ever more important, many of the original functions of the epidermis are transferred to other tissues, or are restricted to areas where control is more easily exercised. Some of these developments are described elsewhere in this book (Chapter 4). The function of the epidermis to act as a barrier between the internal and external environments now becomes of correspondingly greater importance, and the epidermis itself shows adaptations which enable species to live in widely differing habitats. It is perhaps not surprising that the two major animal groups—the arthropods and the vertebrates—which dominate aquatic and terrestrial environments show the greatest development of epidermal adaptations which enable them to live successfully in the most diverse habitats.

Epidermis in invertebrates

In most invertebrates, there is a differentiated single layered epithelium covering the surface of the body although in the chaetognathes the epithelium may be multilayered in parts, resembling the condition characteristic of the vertebrate phyla. In the acoele turbellarians, there is little differentiation between the epidermis and the internal parenchyma, the epidermis lacking a basal membrane and without any underlying network of cutaneous muscles. This condition may be considered primitive. In other turbellarians, the apical parts of the cells fuse into a smooth epithelial layer, the basal ends of the cells remaining independent and embedded in the underlying tissue. In the nemertines, the epithelial cells have broad apical parts which form a smooth layer; the basal outgrowths are branched and the spaces between the branches are filled with glandular, nerve and supporting cells.

The epidermal layer protects the internal environment of the animal from the penetration of harmful substances, and also the loss of useful materials from within. Products of the epidermis can also help the animal to withstand mechanical contacts and even the ravages of predators. In many invertebrates, the epidermis and its products mould the form of the species—unlike the vertebrates, where general body form is determined by the endoskeleton, epidermal derivatives adding only the finer details to specific morphology.

In the coelenterates, turbellarians, nemertines, annelids and molluscs, the secretions of cutaneous mucous and protein glands play a large part in the protective functions of the epidermis. The secretions can become specialized, forming, for example, the rhabdites of turbellarians and the nematocysts of coelenterates. The particularly successful functions of nematocysts have been utilized by animals other than coelenterates, which use them for their own predation and defence. Thus a small number of turbellarians possess nematocysts in their epidermis, derived from ingested hydroids, and used for the capture of prey. Nudibranch molluscs also utilize ingested nematocysts, storing them in special ectodermal sacs, the cnidosacs, containing a diverticulum of the gut. Some nemertines contain nematocysts in the anterior proboscis epithelium: their origin is unknown.

The epidermal mucous secretions may help in locomotion, as in, for example, terrestrial turbellarians, molluscs and nemertines. There is often enhanced secretion of mucus on irritation, injury or exposure to unfavourable conditions. Some freshwater animals may survive the drying up of their habitat by enclosing themselves in mucous cysts, as, for example, the nemertine *Prostoma*. This points the way to another important protective function of epidermal secretions—their solidification to form structures external to the animal.

In the hydroid coelenterates, the epidermis secretes a laminated horny perisarc which acts as a protective external skeleton. When the perisarc is fully formed, the epidermis retreats from beneath it, with connections maintained only at irregular intervals. In some hydroids, the polyps are protected by the cup-like hydrothecae into which they can retreat; reproductive zooids are similarly protected by gonothecae. The calcareous or horny skeletons of corals, providing support as well as protection, although topographically internal in appearance, are, in fact, morphologically external, secreted by the ectoderm.

The polychaete worms show a range of development of protective tubes. Some, such as that produced by *Perinereis*, are simply mucus-lined burrows in mud or sand. In others, such as that of *Pectinaria*, mucus is used to cement together sand grains or pieces of shell. In *Sabella*, ventral sacs beneath the mouth store suitable sand grains, and glands in the sac walls pour out mucus. At the junction of the peristomial collar, a rope of mucus with embedded sand is formed, adding to the tube as the worm slowly rotates within. In the spirorbids, two large glands beneath the collar produce a mucoid substance containing calcium carbonate. The carbonate precipitates out to form the very hard calcareous tube.

Although many molluscs possess epidermal mucus or protein secreting cells, the great characteristic of the phylum is the ability to secrete a shell. The mantle epithelium produces the shell by secretion from special cells at its edge, thus allowing growth at its periphery. As well as the clearly protective function of the shell, it also serves as support for the mantle itself. Most modern molluscs have shells composed of a keratin-like substance, conchiolin, together with calcium carbonate layers. In the aplacophoran molluscs, a shell is absent but the vermiform body is covered by a cuticular mantle in which are embedded calcareous spicules. The polyplacophorans (chitons) have a dorsal armour of eight articulated plates, composed of an outer layer of conchiolin impregnated with calcium carbonate and an inner layer of carbonate alone. The scaphopods have a tapering cylindrical shell, open at both ends, which protects the body during burrowing. The gastropod shell is typically spiral and usually conical. It is first secreted by the larval shell gland as a protoconch and this is represented in the adult by the tip of the spiral cone of the shell. The shells may be elongated and tapering, or flattened and planospiral, or the later formed whorls may completely enclose the earlier ones. A very few gastropods, for example, *Tamanovalva limax* from Japan, have developed a bivalved shell, the spiral protoconch remaining on one shell. In some gastropods, the shell may become reduced in size and covered by the mantle, as in pteropods and some slugs, or else is completely absent as in the nudibranchs. Typically the bivalve molluscs are compressed laterally with a mantle which secretes a single shell of two lobes and a ligament which joins them dorsally at a hinge. Here the shell consists of an outer organic layer, the periostracum, and two crystalline layers of calcium carbonate embedded in an organic matrix. It is interesting that the bivalved condition has also been adopted by other phyla: in the brachiopods the valves are dorsal and ventral, and not lateral as in the bivalved molluscs; some crustaceans (ostracods) have also modified the carapace to resemble the bivalved condition. In the cephalopod molluscs, the shell is external, many chambered, and coiled or straight in the living and fossil nautiloids; but is reduced or absent in the squids and octopods.

Molluscan and brachiopod shells, together with the protective tubes of annelids, are produced by only parts of the epidermal surfaces of the animals. They are thus to be distinguished from cuticles, which are secreted by the epidermal cells overall. Cuticle development is related to the loss of ciliation. Thus cuticle is absent in turbellarians, but is well formed in parasitic flatworms. The cuticle is of considerable thickness in the nematodes, and can be moulted as the animals grow. In *Ascaris*, the cuticle is made up of three main regions composed of nine separate layers. The surface of the cuticle is covered by a very thin, probably lipid, layer. The main outer region is the cortex, formed of keratin perhaps with additional collagen. The middle layer consists of a fibrillar region lying upon a homogeneous layer of albumen-like proteins together with fibroin- or elastin-like fibrous proteins. The innermost layer is made up of three regions of fibres, composed probably of collagen. The fibre layers cross each other to make up a system of minute parallelograms. The fibres are inextensible but they allow stretching and shortening of the cuticle by their relative movement upon each other. The structure of the cuticle is of considerable importance in allowing body movements during locomotion and other functions.

In the bryozoans, the cuticle forms the external skeleton of the zooids: it may be membranous, chitinous, gelatinous or have additional calcification. The frontal wall of the zooid is uncalcified in some bryozoans, leaving a window covered by a flexible membrane. Muscles attached to this membrane can pull it inwards, increasing the hydrostatic pressure of the coelom and so causing the evagination of the introvert with its tentacles.

The best developed cuticle is found in the arthropods. It consists essentially of two parts: an outer epicuticle and an inner endocuticle. The epicuticle in most arthropods is two layered, the inner layer composed of a lipoprotein complex which may be tanned (see below) and an outer lipoid or wax layer. In some arthropod groups, the wax layer itself may be covered by a secretion from the dermal glands, the cement layer, which may be similar to shellac in composition. The epicuticle does not contain the polysaccharide chitin, but chitin is characteristically present in the endocuticle of all arthropods. The endocuticle is a layered structure composed of a mixture of chitin and proteins, the latter generically termed arthropodin. In the outer layers of parts of the endocuticle, the protein chains are joined together by polyphenol derivatives to form a tough, resistant compound called sclerotin. The process of joining the protein molecules is termed sclerotization or tanning. The tergal and sternal plates are the most obvious regions of sclerotization, together with the head capsule and joints of the limbs. The cuticle may be calcified as well as tanned, as in many crustaceans. The net result of tanning, giving hard sclerotized regions alternating with untanned cuticle, is to produce a highly flexible, articulating exoskeleton, which not only supports the body and provides bases for the attachment of muscles, but also enables complex locomotory and other movements to be performed.

Epidermis in terrestrial invertebrates

Colonization of the land presents the epithelium with a new problem—prevention of evaporation of body water from the organism, and at the same time to allow respiratory gas exchange which has to take place across a moist surface film. In many terrestrial invertebrates the problem has not been solved and the animals are not completely emancipated from their aquatic origins. Thus land planarians largely inhabit the forest floor of tropical and subtropical jungles; they require high humidities and remain concealed under stones, logs and leaf mould during the day. The terrestrial nematodes live in the water films around soil particles, vegetation, etc., and in this sense could be considered still to be aquatic. Under desiccating conditions, many nematodes can withstand a certain degree of drying out, and enter a state of anabiosis, becoming active again when water is once more available. In spite of these apparent limitations to a fully terrestrial life, the numbers of nematodes, both in terms of species and of individuals, suggest highly successful exploitation of their particular habitats.

Earthworms are able to lose 75% of their total body water without dying, although under natural conditions, behavioural reactions to seek higher humidities are induced long before this percentage loss occurs. The normal environment of an earthworm is between that of a freshwater animal and that of an air dweller, and many species avoid waterlogged situations—which perhaps explains why they leave their burrows after heavy rains.

In the examples given above, respiration takes place over the whole surface of the animals, and no provision can be made for the protection of this respiratory surface. The animals are all related to freshwater forms, and it is to be supposed that terrestrial migration occurred *via* fresh waters.

With terrestrial molluscs, the evidence points to a direct invasion of the land from the sea. The land forms comprise the pulmonate gastropods (snails and slugs) together with representatives of four main prosobranch superfamilies, the operculate land snails. These diverse groups show parallel evolution in structural development, including the replacement of gills in the mantle cavity by a vascularized region, the lung. In land snails, the control of water loss is a major physiological problem and consequently high environmental humidities are essential. However, 100% relative humidity is not necessarily the optimum for all species: evaporation of water from the body surface has a cooling effect, and enables body temperatures to be maintained at a level below that of the environment. Consequently, a low relative humidity allows survival at quite high environmental temperatures providing that the exposure times are relatively short. Moreover, the land snails can reduce water loss considerably by withdrawing into their shells; slugs do not have this choice, but they can withstand water losses up to 50% of their body weight.

Like the molluscs, terrestrial crustaceans have also colonized the land *via* the sea shore. The terrestrial isopods (woodlice) have close relatives living high up on the shore, and structurally they closely resemble the marine forms. Many crabs and hermit crabs show various degrees of adaptation to a terrestrial environment: the hermit crab, *Birgus latro*, is perhaps the most land-adapted of all the decapods, although it still has a marine larval stage and therefore cannot be considered as emancipated from the sea as are the woodlice.

In marine decapods, the gills are protected by the lateral walls of the carapace. This protection is retained in the semi-terrestrial and terrestrial forms, but now provides a certain degree of protection from water loss as well as the original protection from mechanical damage and shock. There is, however, a progressive reduction in the number of gills, or gill volume in relation to body volume, related to the degree of emancipation from water. Associated with this is the development of vascular tufts and vascularization in the roof or walls of the gill chambers, best formed in *Birgus* which also has blood lacunae in the dorsal abdominal wall. The replacement of gills by lungs in terrestrial crabs thus parallels the similar development in terrestrial molluscs.

In *Birgus*, ventilation of the respiratory chamber occurs partly by movements of the scaphognathite—which thus has a function in moving air exactly similar to that for moving water in aquatic forms. But in *Birgus*, ventilation also occurs by movements of the pleural margins of the carapace, which are raised by special muscles not found in purely aquatic species. In the woodlice, the pleopods are respiratory as they are in the marine isopods, but in some species, some or all of the exopodites possess hollow tuft-like invaginations—the pseudotracheae. The species with pseudotracheae have the advantage that they are less subject to oxygen lack in dry air than those without.

In dry air, a motionless slug can lose by transpiration about 2·5% of its original weight per hour; this increases to about 16% per hour if the slug is continually stimulated to move. In semi-terrestrial crabs, the rate varies from about 0·25% to 0·65% of the original weight per hour. Direct comparisons between slugs and crabs cannot be made because surface area to volume relationships are of the greatest importance in determining transpiration rates. However, the difference in transpiration rates between the two groups is so great that overall it may be surmised that the calcified crustacean exoskeleton does confer a certain degree of impermeability upon the semi- and fully-terrestrial forms. But in spite of this, the problem of water loss is still of the greatest importance to the land crustaceans, and they are hence usually cryptozoic in their behaviour. The cooling effects of transpiration in land crustaceans, as in the terrestrial molluscs, allow the animals to survive environmental temperatures close to their thermal death points providing the relative humidity is low and the exposure short; the upper lethal temperatures are considerably lower at long exposures and low relative humidities because the beneficial effects of transpiration are counterbalanced by rapid desiccation.

In the ticks, spiders, scorpions, and particularly the insects, there is a wax-like layer in the epicuticle which confers major waterproofing properties upon the integuments of these animals. In the centipedes and millipedes, it has been suggested that the dermal glands secrete a lipoid material which forms a film and confers some degree of water-proofing upon the cuticle, which varies according to the species. In the insects, the wax layer may have the consistency of a soft grease or be of varying degrees of hardness. The wax molecules are randomly orientated except for a monolayer of orientated molecules next to the cuticle. The arrangement of molecules in the monolayer is such that it is impermeable to water, but at a 'critical temperature', determined by the nature of the wax according to species, thermal agitation disrupts the organized monolayer and permeability to water increases sharply at this temperature.

Some terrestrial arthropods, including some insects, have the additional property of being able to take up water through their cuticles from sub-saturated atmospheres. The mechanism by which this is achieved is unknown, but it does serve to accentuate the remarkable control of water balance developed in the fully terrestrial arthropods, not only in relation to the properties of the epidermis and its secretions, but in many other aspects of their metabolism, morphology and behaviour. The development of the wax layer in particular enables insects and the arachnomorphs to be as completely adapted for terrestrial life as the reptiles, birds and mammals amongst the vertebrates.

Epidermis in vertebrates

A characteristic feature of the vertebrate epidermis from the most primitive fish to the higher tetrapods is its stratified appearance imparted by the several layers of cells. In lower vertebrates the basal germinal layer has a multiplicity of functions in that it can give rise to cells which probably secrete mucin, glandular cells and sensory receptors. By contrast, in higher tetrapods, the potential of the cells is restricted to keratin formation, glandular cells for the most part being confined to the epidermal appendages. Also receptor cells whilst taking origin in the epidermal layer have in higher vertebrates become relatively remote from it and grouped for the most part in the dermis.

CYCLOSTOMES

Amongst the cyclostomates (the hagfishes and lampreys—the most primitive jawless vertebrates) the epidermis is very thick and multi-layered. The epidermis contains cuticle forming cells and large glandular cells which discharge their contents when they reach the skin surface. The hagfish has in addition to glandular cells a series of mucous glands which are epidermal in origin but located in the dermis. The contents of these glands can be forcibly ejected when the animal is disturbed and form a viscous secretion which can transform the surrounding water into jelly-like consistency. These glands which are under neural control are thought to provide the hagfish with protection against ectoparasites. As in all vertebrates the epidermis extends into the oral cavity but in cyclostomes small epidermal teeth are found which are not true teeth but are highly keratinized horny derivatives of the epithelium.

ELASMOBRANCH FISHES

In the elasmobranchs (sharks, rays, skates and chimaeras) the epidermis contains scattered sensory cells in addition to numerous glandular goblet cells and a third type of cell, which produces the fine cuticular layer, which although difficult to observe, probably occurs in these as in all fish. The surface of the skin is characterized by denticles of dermal origin but the epidermis contributes to the new emerging core of the denticle a layer of very hard crystalline enamel which has a very low organic content when compared with the deeper layer, the dentine. As the denticle thus formed reaches the surface of the skin it pierces the epidermis to give the rough texture of the body surface.

GANOID FISHES

In the actinopterygians (ganoid fishes) it has been suggested that the base of the epidermal layer may secrete a protein into the basal lamina which acts as a focal point for crystallization of the dermal scales. As in the elasmobranchs there is here also the possibility that the epidermis also contributes to the scale formation.

TELEOST FISHES

In teleosts (bony fishes) the epidermis contains cuticle forming cells as well as glandular and sensory cells, the whole forming a continuous surface layer over the scales which, relatively speaking, are reduced to thin flexible collagenous plates rich in calcium salts. The actual surface of bony fish is cuticular although this is rarely seen; it is, however, uniquely thick in the sea horse (*Hippocampus*).

The cuticle which extends over the whole surface of the body and the oral and gill surfaces is sloughed periodically, probably to allow for general body growth. This cyclic activity may be under hormonal control. Specialized structures of epidermal origin include the modified epidermal cells which form electric storage plates (in the electric catfish), keratinization of the horny lips of certain herbivorous fish and the breeding tubercles of some inshore marine teleosts and some freshwater teleosts are also formed from keratinization of localized areas of the epidermis. The expanded epithelial covering of the gills contain specialized secretory cells called chloride cells to which has been attributed a specialist role in electrolyte exchange with the environment; a view which now finds little support (see p. 57).

While the majority of the nerves supplying the integument terminate in the deep dermis and sub-epidermal layers, nerve endings are found in the epidermis terminating on spindle-shaped receptor cells. Certain receptors found in the epidermis of *Pomatochiatus* are similar in appearance to the taste cells of mammals and function as chemoreceptors.

In animals cushioned in the constancy of an aquatic environment, sensitivity to changes in their physical environment is of paramount importance. In the fish and the more aquatic amphibians is developed the lateralis sensory system supplied by the VII, IX and X cranial nerves. Two different types of organs are found. First, there is in lungfishes, elasmobranchs and ganoids the ampullary organ consisting of pits in the epidermis lined with receptor cells. The cavity of the pit contains a jelly-like substance characterized by high electrical conductivity. These pits are distributed widely over the head and enable fish to orientate in an electric field. Of greater importance is the neuromast system which enables fish to register water movement and vibrations; a system which has obvious advantages in the animal's appreciation of environmental change and bears particular importance during shoaling. In many ways their system resembles the labyrinth of the inner ear of mammals and indeed is an evolutionary forerunner of this part of the ear. Because of this the lateralis system is frequently referred to as the acoustico-lateralis system.

Amphibians

Amphibians are remarkable in the diversity of habitats they occupy. They range from the purely aquatic toad (*Xenopus*) to those which survive the most hostile arid condition (*Chiroleptes, Cyclorana*). No amphibian is, however, completely adapted to terrestrial life for the larval stages are always aquatic so that the adults return to water for breeding. Even those found in the desert avoid the extremes of the environment through behavioural characteristics which ensure protection from desiccation as a result of prolonged exposure to sunlight (see p. 60). Amphibian epidermal cells have importance as sites of electrolyte balance (pp. 14, 57) and of course are important in many cases as extensive and additional respiratory surfaces. Amphibians resemble fish in that in their larval stages the epidermis is unkeratinized and covered with a fine cuticle and the larvae develop horny teeth resembling the cyclostome situation (see above). In contrast the metamorphosed adult epidermis is keratinized, although to varying degrees. Despite this the skin serves as an efficient respiratory organ in aquatic forms and to this end there is found in the much folded surface a close proximity of the fine vascular network, facilitating the easy exchange of respiratory gases. These epidermal blood capillaries are found in those species which have persistent larval stages. In the more terrestrial representatives, the epidermis of the larva comprising larval cuticle and epidermal cells, sloughs at metamorphosis and the cells underneath secrete a new cuticle which becomes keratinized as it reaches the surface. The horny layer is periodically sloughed, temperature being the main determinant, sloughing occurring more frequently at higher temperatures.

The skin of amphibians contains numerous glands. Principal amongst these are the mucous glands which provide the moisture for the skin, enabling it to function as a respiratory surface. In those amphibians with dry skin, mucous cells also occur but they are much fewer in number: in such examples the additional respiratory surface is provided through the buccal cavity. Mucous glands which are controlled by the nervous system are usually accompanied by other glands whose secretion is poisonous when released, serving as a deterrent to potential predators.

Reptiles

The reptiles were the first vertebrates to successfully colonize and become adapted to life on land. They achieved this by virtue of their independence from water during early development, by the abandonment of the skin as a respiratory surface and by the increase in concentrating capacity of the kidneys. The glandular components of the epidermis tend to be concentrated in specialized glands and the keratinized epidermis is much thickened and undergoes periodic sloughing; a process largely under the control of the hormones thyroxine and prolactin.

Birds

The avian skin displays many reptilian characters but is distinctive because of a new epidermal appendage, the feather, a structure derived from the reptilian epidermal scale. The feathers serve a multiplicity of functions, principally as a resistant, protective and waterproof covering, and through the trapping of air in dead spaces, as an insulatory system. The only important skin gland is the uropygial gland or preen gland which produces an oil which assists in the water-proofing of the feather. Not all birds have this gland but it is particularly well developed in those birds which actually alight on water. There are various types of feathers the detailing of which is outside the scope of this book. It is important to realize however that the feather cycle of growth culminates in a moult and the evidence suggests that the moult is controlled by hormones. As discussed elsewhere (p. 155) colour in birds is important both in camouflage and as a part of the process whereby the sexes are brought together.

Mammals

In mammals the characteristic epidermal appendage is the hair which serves many of the functions described for feathers, e.g. heat conservation, colour protection. They are, however, phylogenetically quite distinct from feathers. Hair growth and replacement occurs in cycles. Many mammals moult twice a year usually in spring and autumn, for example, lemming and hare. Such an arrangement provides a long coat for the inclement winter and a short coat for the less hostile times of the year. Other animals have only one moult—spring in the common seal and autumn in the northern fur seal. The evidence suggests that the onset of moult is determined by environmental cues, principally the lengthening of daylight in spring and the shortening in the autumn. These environmental events are translated into changes in the endocrinology of these animals via their detection on the retina, from which afferent pathways connect to the hypothalamus of the brain to regulate the output of hypothalamic releasing factors, which in turn modify the release of pituitary tropic hormones. This sequence of physiological events alters the production of the endocrine secretions which exert their effect directly on the hair follicles. The mechanism is complex but oestrogens, testosterone, glucocorticoids and thyroxine have all been implicated.

Mammals are unique in the possession of specialized glands called sweat glands. These have their greatest physiological importance in the naked human skin where continuous evaporation from a hair-free surface is an efficient mechanism of water loss. Such a continuous process in animals with a thick pelt would contribute little to thermoregulation, for in such cases the fur would merely become wet and evaporation from the surface of the pelt would have little effect. In animals with pelts, therefore, sweating over the body surface is confined to single short periods of sweat formation coincident with periods of extreme muscular activity, such as when escaping from predators. Small mammals on the other hand have sweat glands confined to the foot pads, and heat loss is achieved by panting and vasodilation of the less covered parts of the body. Sweat is an important route of Na^+ loss from the body, but this loss is minimized in the Na^+ depleted animal through the reabsorption of this ion by the action of the adrenal hormone, aldosterone. This hormone is, of course, of major importance in the control of electrolyte balance in the nephron (see p. 51).

Chapter 4
Excretory Organs

General considerations

Waste products leave the bodies of animals in many ways. For example, water may leave by the skin, from the lungs, the urine and in the faeces. Carbon dioxide is lost mainly by the lungs, but also appears in urine and sweat as bicarbonate ions. Calcium and magnesium leave the vertebrate body in both urine and faeces, the relative balance between the two routes varying greatly between species.

There is no concise chemical definition of excretion; it is best defined in a general way as the separation and elimination from the body of metabolic wastes. Some compounds may be excretory products at one time but may be metabolically useful at others. For example, water, carbon dioxide and ammonia can be subjected to a variety of treatments depending upon the needs of the animal. Water which forms as a by-product of metabolism may be the only source of water for some animals and is thus conserved. However, water has often to be removed, when present in large amounts, to prevent osmotic flooding of the tissues. Both carbon dioxide and ammonia are necessary building blocks for some anabolic processes, though more generally they are waste products of metabolism and removed from the body.

No special excretory organs have been described for the majority of protozoa, sponges and coelenterates. The fact that these are small animals affords them no special protection against their environment. For example, freshwater protozoa can be faced with serious osmotic flooding. It must be remembered that as linear dimensions are reduced the ratio of surface area/unit volume increases so that small animals have relatively large surface areas. Unless the permeability of the cell membrane has been correspondingly reduced, they will have to excrete relatively more water than larger animals. In most of the organisms within the above groups, the unmodified cell membrane can cope with this problem. However, all freshwater protozoa and sponges have specialized organs, contractile vacuoles, which function primarily as a means of evacuating this excess water. It is possible that the contractile vacuole has become modified so that waste products are secreted into it but this aspect of its function is probably secondary to its osmotic function. The waste products being expelled from the body when the vacuole contracts to push out the water. Thus the contractile vacuole probably functions also as an excretory organ.

Waste products of metabolism are not always removed from the body, they can be stored either temporarily or permanently within special regions. For example, many insects and spiders, even though they possess well-developed and functional excretory tubes, store their excretory products in specialized cells and tissues. However, in the springtails, arthropods which lack Malpighian tubes (see following section), all their waste nitrogen, which is in the form of uric acid, is stored. Earthworms possess well-developed and functional excretory tubes termed nephridia (see following section), but the epithelium surrounding the gut and blood vessels is also modified into special excretory tissue, the chloragen cells. Some of the metabolic waste extracted from the blood is thought to accumulate within these cells, which finally become detached and float in the coelomic fluid. This fluid contains amoeboid cells which ingest detached chloragen cells and finally deposit the waste under the body wall. Some degenerated chloragen cells are lost via the nephridia.

Nephridia and coelomoducts

In morphological terms, the nature of excretory organs varies from group to group. Apart from the unspecialized surface of the body which may be utilized as in the protozoans and the coelenterates, specialized epithelial coverings may be developed, as in gills and the sweat glands of the skin.

Many invertebrates have a structure termed the nephridium which has an intracellular lumen terminating in the body cavity (coelom) as a special cellular structure, the flame cell or solenocyte (Fig. 4.1A). At its other end, the nephridium may either open into the body cavity (metanephridia) or to the exterior (protonephridia). The respective openings are termed nephridiostomes and nephridiopores. Nephridia are found in platyhelminths, rotifers, annelids and molluscs.

Excretion of fluids from the coelom takes place by way of paired structures termed coelomoducts. In contrast with nephridia, coelomoducts have an intercellular lumen and no flame cell. They are found in annelids, molluscs, arthropods, echinoderms and chordates. It is customary to consider the various kinds of nephridia as homologous. Similarly, coelomoducts in the various groups are thought to be homologous, with a probable origin as genital ducts to convey eggs and sperm to the exterior, whereas now they also assist in excretion.

In some organisms, notably the polychaetes, both nephridium and coelomoduct are closely linked, forming a compound organ called the nephromixium. This structure may either be concerned both with genital and excretory functions, or may be excretory only.

With regard to the exact function of these invertebrate excretory organs, little is known because of the difficulties in carrying out chemical analysis of fluids in microscopical quantities. The antennary gland of the crayfish which consists of a complex nephridial structure has however been extensively studied. Essentially, it is a coiled tube with a complicated sac at one end and a bladder opening to the exterior at the other (Fig. 4.1B). The coelosac and the labyrinth at the proximal end contain fluid with a composition identical to that of the

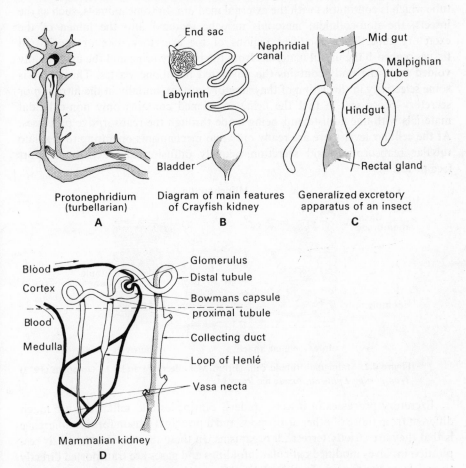

Figure 4.1. Excretory tubules.

blood, except that it contains no proteins. Passing along the coiled nephridial canal, the tubular fluid decreases in concentration until in the bladder, the contents are only about 5% as concentrated as in the coelomosac. The nephridial canal is not found in marine crustaceans, and since the copious fluid released from the gland in crayfish is very low in salt, it is assumed that the nephridium is concerned with the removal of water that enters the body by osmosis and has the capacity to actively remove waste salts from the primary urine.

All excretory tube systems exhibit the same physiological phenomena of filtration or secretion of body fluid to produce a primary urine and then subsequent reabsorption of the filtered or secreted fluid to give the final urine which is voided. In filtration, use is made of hydrostatic pressure to filter non-colloidal materials from the body fluids and pass them into the lumen of the excretory tube which is continuous with the external medium. In some animals, such as the insects, the non-colloidal materials may be secreted into the lumen of the excretory tube. Then modified regions of the excretory tube or specialized tissues reabsorb the useful materials from the primary urine and the urine finally voided from the body contains the unwanted metabolic wastes. Thus there is some selectivity in the action of the excretory system, initially in the filtration or secretory processes, in that the urine so formed contains only non-colloidal materials with fine adjustments being made through the reabsorptive processes. At the cellular level there are really only two mechanisms operating to regulate tubular reabsorption and secretion, namely diffusion and active transport (see p. 12).

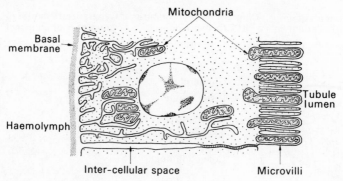

Figure 4.2. Malpighian tubule cell. (From M.J. Berridge and J.L. Oschman (1972) *Transporting Epithelia*, Academic Press.)

Excretory processes in insects, spiders, centipedes and millipedes are much different from those of other arthropods and a principal reason for this difference is that they are strictly terrestrial organisms. In these terrestrial arthropods respiration involves modified cuticular infoldings and gases are transported directly to and from the tissues. The blood (in this case haemolymph) is not circulated around the body under pressure. Thus although these organisms have excretory tubes their function is in no way dependent upon blood pressure. The excretory system of an insect is shown in Fig. 4.1C, and consists of Malpighian tubes and the hindgut. The tubes, which open into the gut at the junction between the mid- and hindguts, are closed at their distal ends and hang free in the haemolymph. Excretion through the Malpighian tubes is by secretion into the lumen of an isosmotic solution of low molecular weight compounds from the haemolymph (Fig. 4.2). The basal and apical surfaces of the Malpighian tubule cells are highly infolded and the mitochondria are often associated with these infoldings. Urine flow is probably initiated by local osmotic gradients established in the narrow channels present between the infoldings of the basal membrane and the apical microvilli. These gradients could be formed by the active secretion of ions; water then being drawn through the basement membrane along an osmotic gradient. The primary urine formed in this way contains much more potassium than sodium and it is the active secretion of potassium which is the prime factor in initiating urine flow. Amino acids, sugars and waste materials are carried with this fluid flow (Fig. 4.3). There is a continuous flow into the hindgut of this

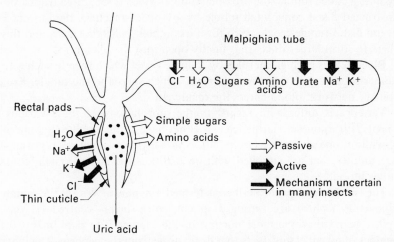

Figure 4.3. Water and solute transport through the Malpighian tube and rectal pads. Insoluble uric acid precipitated in the hindgut is excreted.

isosmotic urine (the rate of flow may vary considerably; see p. 94) but the final composition of the urine voided from the insect depends upon the reabsorptive powers of the rectal pads and the hindgut epithelium (see p. 92).

Kidney

Many workers use the term kidney to describe the antennary gland in the crayfish and it does incorporate the three basic features of the vertebrate kidney; namely, a closed proximal structure through which the body fluid passes to produce a protein-free ultrafiltrate, a convoluted tubule in which the salt and water content of the filtrate are modified, and a storage organ at the distal end, which opens through the exterior surface of the body.

Kidneys proper are confined to the vertebrates and although they vary in structure according to evolutionary level, are always constructed on the same general plan, consisting of a mass of coelomoducts opening into a single longitudinal collecting duct. Depending on its complexity the structure is termed a mesonephros in fishes and amphibia, and a metanephros, of somewhat different origin, in the amniotes.

In mammals, the original openings of the coelomoducts to the coelom have been lost and each begins embryologically as a blind enlargement of the tubule termed the Bowman's capsule (Fig. 4.1D). A cavity develops in this capsule into which a bundle of blood capillaries, derived from the renal artery, is inserted. This capillary bed, called the glomerulus, and the Bowman's capsule are collectively known as the Malpighian body. Distally, the Bowman's capsule becomes a coiled tubule (the proximal tubule) which is separated from a similarly constructed distal convoluted tubule by a looped structure, the loop of Henlé. Several distal tubules coalesce to form a common collecting duct, and this joins others to form larger ducts that finally open into the bladder.

Blood leaves each glomerulus by a single vessel which then branches to form another set of capillaries, the vasa recta, which surround the tubule. From this capillary network, blood enters the renal vein.

Vertebrates differ with regard to the morphology of these various components; for example, marine teleosts either have a much reduced glomerulus or are without one altogether (see p. 50). Animals possessing a renal portal system have tubules that are supplied with an additional capillary system containing venous blood.

The tubular unit just described is termed a nephron. Within the mammalian kidney the nephroi are arranged in concentric layers centred on the renal papilla; being the innermost portion of the kidney. The papilla supports the openings of all collecting ducts that drain urine from the nephroi. The inner zone of the kidney (medulla) contains the loop of Henlé, and parts of the collecting ducts, whereas the outer zone (cortex) contains glomeruli, and the proximal and distal tubules.

In other vertebrate kidneys, loops of Henlé are not found and the layering of tubules is not so well defined. Also, the general shape of the organ differs, ranging from the long, thin linearly arranged kidneys of fish to the lobular kidneys of birds. Bird kidneys may possess a complex tubular structure functionally equivalent to the loop of Henlé.

The mechanisms by which the plasma filtrate is converted into urine are not fully understood, but the basic features have been assessed. From studies in which small samples of fluid were removed directly from the tubules, it appears that the contents of the proximal tubule are similar in composition to a fluid which can be obtained from the blood by dialysis. The major difference between this tubular fluid and plasma is that it contains no proteins. Therefore, the membrane of the Malpighian body must be impermeable to proteins. From a comparison of the two solutions, it would be expected that fluid would pass back from the tubular fluid to the plasma by osmosis because of the colloid osmotic pressure deficit in the tubule. In fact, the tubular fluid moves down the tubule away from Bowman's capsule, and this can only happen if a hydrostatic pressure exists across the glomerular membrane. This pressure is maintained by the heart. Experimentally, it has been observed that when the arterial pressure falls below 40 mm of mercury, secretion of urine ceases; the colloid osmotic pressure due to proteins in the blood is about 30 mm Hg.

Secretion of urine may also be stopped experimentally by placing a ligature on the ureter; urine ceases to be formed when the pressure in the water is about 90 mm Hg and that in the arteries about 130 mm. The difference of about 40 mm Hg is clearly the maximum pressure available for forcing water and small molecules through the blood capillaries into the tubule.

Using the frog as an experimental animal, it is possible by using micropipettes to remove and measure all the fluid entering a single Bowman's capsule. Since the total number of capsules can be estimated, the rate of filtration of plasma may be calculated and compared with the rate of urine formation. Filtration occurs at a rate that is about ten times that of urine production, so that about 90% of the filtrate must be reabsorbed as it passes down the nephron. As many of the constituents of blood plasma do not differ markedly in respect to their concentrations in urine, despite the massive reabsorption of water, they must also be reabsorbed.

The early researchers into kidney function placed substances in two divisions according to the way in which they were regulated during their passage through the nephron. Substances that were completely absorbed, unless the concentration in the blood was increased above a 'normal' value were termed 'threshold substances'; the assumption being that if the level in the tubule increased above a critical value, the cells lining the walls would not be able to absorb them fast enough. The classical substance in this group is glucose. The other class of 'no-threshold' substances included those molecules that are not absorbed and are always excreted no matter what level they reach in the blood. Because of the large proportion of water reabsorbed, these 'no-threshold' substances would always show an increased concentration, comparing plasma with urine. Although it is now thought that very few substances belong to the 'no-threshold' class, the old distinction is useful in relation to the role of the kidney in allowing substances in excess of the body's need to be excreted.

Tubules also have the capacity to add substances to the filtrate. Powerful evidence for this function comes from the observation that increasing the rate of filtration does not have an equal effect on the amounts of all excretory products, as would be expected if the kidney did nothing but absorb indiscriminately. For example, a greatly increased filtration rate in man has very little effect on the net excretion of ammonia, sulphate and phosphate. A likely explanation of this result is that these substances must be in part secreted by the tubules at a constant rate.

Detailed analysis of the composition of mammalian tubular fluid indicates that about 75% of the filtrate is reabsorbed by the time the fluid enters the loop of Henlé. Experimental evidence shows also that there is a steady increase in osmotic pressure of the kidney tissue from cortex to the innermost part of the medulla, and this is thought to indicate the operation of concentrating mechanisms on the contents of the nephrons. This osmotic pressure gradient is thought to be induced through differences in the permeability of tubules to water and sodium, together with variations in sodium transport as follows.

Water, Na^+ and Cl^+ pass freely through the walls of the descending limbs of the loop of Henlé (Fig. 4.4). As the tubular fluid enters the lower regions of the medulla, which have a higher osmotic pressure, water is withdrawn osmotically and sodium ions tend to enter with an appropriate anion to maintain the osmotic

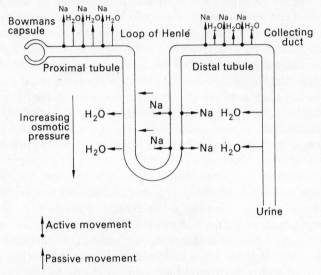

Figure 4.4. Urine formation in the mammalian kidney.

pressure close to that existing outside the tubule. It is not so easy for Na^+ and water to pass through the walls of the first part of the ascending limb. However, the cells lining the tubule actively transport Na^+ out into the extracellular tissues. As a result, the tubular fluid becomes progressively more dilute as it passes up the loop, due to the loss of a fluid high in Na^+ and low in water, and may come to have a lower osmotic pressure than plasma.

It is envisaged that much of the Na^+ removed from the ascending loop enters the descending loop and the high osmotic pressure of the medulla is maintained by this recycling process.

The walls of the distal tubule are thought to be freely permeable to water, and it is assumed that no further reduction in fluid volume occurs in this region once the tubular fluid has become isosmotic with plasma, although there may be further selective active uptake of sodium ions. The final stage of concentration takes place in the collecting ducts.

The rate and pattern of blood flow within the Bowman's capsule and the tubules would also be expected to play an important role in the regulation of both filtration and reabsorption. With regard to filtration, there is evidence that urine composition is influenced by changes in blood pressure at the level of the glomerulus, and the rate of removal of intercellular electrolytes is also regulated by variations in the rate and pattern of blood flow through the peritubular blood vessels (the vasa recta).

Alterations in the blood composition, which if unchecked would lead to cellular changes, are regulated by an automatic system for varying the composition of the urine. An antidiuretic hormone (ADH), produced in the hypothalamus but released from the posterior lobe of the pituitary gland, and aldosterone from the adrenal cortex, are released in response to changes in the salt and water content of the blood. In the hypothalamus and parts of the vascular system these changes are registered by groups of specialized cells, which are able to detect very small variations in Na^+ concentration, osmotic pressure and mechanical pressure of the blood.

ADH stimulates specifically the process by which water is reabsorbed from the tubule into the tubular cells. The manner in which this is achieved is not understood fully, but it involves a decrease in the permeability barrier to the osmotic movement of water through the cell membranes lining the tubules. If sufficient ADH is administered urine will be produced which is similar in composition to that formed by an individual deprived of drinking water.

The adrenal gland produces hormones that affect the Na^+ conservation processes located in the kidney tubule. Removal of the adrenal glands, an operation called adrenalectomy, results in a low rate of Na^+ uptake by the kidney tubules, an effect which is responsible for the progressive leaching from the body of Na^+ in such animals. If untreated the animal finally succumbs and death follows. The reabsorption of Na^+ can be returned to normal by the administration of an extract of the adrenal cortex. Such extracts contain a variety of steroid hormones, several of which have similar effects on Na^+ reabsorption. Minor variations in molecular structure, however, are associated with large differences in biological activity; that with the greatest activity in respect of Na^+ reabsorption in the kidney is called aldosterone.

Thus aldosterone from the adrenal cortex and antidiuretic hormone from the posterior lobe of the pituitary act in combination on the reabsorptive mechanisms of the kidney to conserve water and salt. This statement is, in fact, an oversimplification of the situation, for these hormones are not wholly responsible for the reabsorptive processes throughout the length of the kidney tubule, but they are the essential agents which provide the fine regulation of water and salt gain (and loss) in the tubule and, therefore control of the composition of the final urine. Under conditions of extreme deprivation of salt and water the volume of urine produced is only reduced by about one third and, under these conditions, there is a limitation also of the quantity of Na^+ which can be reabsorbed by the kidney tubule; all the Na^+ which is filtered is never reabsorbed completely. As a result of this limitation of the reabsorptive processes in man, approximately 3 g of Na^+ dissolved in approximately 500 ml of water is lost unavoidably each twenty-four hours. It follows, therefore, that a shipwrecked person deprived of a supply of fresh water could replace the water lost through the kidneys by drinking 500 ml of sea water. Why is such a course fatal? Each 500 ml of sea water contains about 6 g of Na^+, and although the urinary loss of water would be rectified, the Na^+ content of the body would rise by about 3 g. Thus there would be a progressive accumulation of salt in the body—and this is the main reason why man cannot make good the water losses associated with a diet in which sea water is the sole source of drinking water. The shipwrecked man, in fact, reacts by excreting the excess salt at the highest concentration that the kidneys are capable of producing, but at this concentration the urinary water loss is greater than the volume ingested and severe dehydration results. The manner in which whales, seals, and porpoises are able to survive in their marine environment remains a mystery, because it would appear that they are endowed no better than are humans as far as the concentrating capacity of the kidney is concerned.

Man cannot survive in the desert without a source of fresh water because of the inadequate concentrating power of the kidney, which together with the losses in sweat leads rapidly to dehydration. The inability of man to survive in the exacting environment of arid regions without a source of fresh water is not shared by all mammals, for some—for instance the desert rat (*Dipodomys*)—have successfully colonized the deserts of the earth. These small rodents never drink, and water economy is exercised by reducing the production of urine to minute amounts. The Na^+ concentration of the urine is about six-fold greater than that of plasma. They can therefore obtain sufficient water from their food and from the biological oxidation of foodstuffs to remain in water balance.

In what way, then, do desert rats differ from man? The volume of urine voided is reduced to insignificant amounts because of the almost complete reabsorption of the blood filtrate in the kidney tubule. This is achieved in part by an unusually high concentration of ADH in their blood. This circumstance is thought to facilitate the reabsorption of a larger number of water molecules for each Na^+ ion 'pumped' than in the case of man; a condition which is also necessary for the greatly increased concentration of urinary Na^+. Connected with this hormonal adaptation is the presence of an unusual anatomical feature within the kidneys, in the form of an unusually long loop of Henlé which is thought to increase greatly the concentrating power of the kidney.

The behaviour pattern of desert rats contributes further to the economy of water. They actively avoid heat stress and modify the loss of water from extra-renal sites such as the lungs. Also there is another interesting behavioural adaptation in this species in that they store seeds, which form a major part of the diet, in burrows in which the humidity is high compared with the ambient conditions above ground. In this way the seeds contain a higher percentage of water than would otherwise be the case. Thus we see that both hormonal and non-hormonal factors contribute to the success of desert rats in regions where man is not able to survive without access to water.

The problem of Na^+ excretion is not the only requirement which places a high premium on water demands. The need to eliminate urea requires also the loss of water but the kidney of the desert rat is very efficient in this respect, being able to produce a urine with a concentration of urea as high as 24% (compared with a figure for man of 6%). Thus the desert rat requires only about one fourth as much water to eliminate a given amount of urea as a man would. The phenomenal concentrating capacity of the desert rat kidney would suggest that they could drink sea water. Of course desert rats normally would not be exposed to such a source of drinking water. Schmidt-Nielson, however, induced a group of desert rats to imbibe sea water by feeding them with a high protein diet (soy beans) which resulted in the need to excrete a large amount of urea. This forced the rats to drink in order to avoid dehydration. The animal's kidney proved capable of excreting both the excess urea and salt in the sea water. Thus the drinking of sea water enabled the animal to remain in water balance.

It is possible that the camel's kidney operates with similar efficiency. They are known to drink 'bitter waters' and in coastal regions camels browse on seaweed along the shore line which would have a salt content approaching sea water. Water loss through the kidney is reduced severely during dehydration. For example, a camel subjected to summer heat, loses only about 1 litre of water as urine each day. Another important adaptation in this species is the capacity to protect the vascular compartment at the expense of tissue water. For example, in a young camel which had lost about 50 litres of water as a result of dehydration, only a litre had been lost from the blood volume. The mechanism responsible for the protection of the vascular compartment may involve the phenomenon of urea recycling. Camels and kangaroos both have the capacity to reprocess urea (excreted normally via the kidneys) into new protein. Thus amino acids are converted to urea in the liver as in other mammals but the urea thus formed may return via the blood stream to the stomach where it can be reprocessed into protein by the microbial flora of the rumen. Thus the high concentration of urea in the blood makes it highly hyperosmotic to the tissues and as a result water leaves the tissues to preserve the integrity of the blood compartment. Since urea excretion is reduced a further advantage of this uraemia to desert animals is the saving of urinary water.

Salt glands

Vertebrates other than mammals also face environmental fluctuations that tend to alter the composition of the body fluids. In Chapter 2 it was pointed out that there is a remarkable constancy of Na^+ concentration in body fluids in all vertebrates (with but a few exceptions) and it seems that the hormones concerned principally with the maintenance of this constant concentration are those of the adrenal gland and posterior lobe of the pituitary. In large measure the adrenal hormones are chemically the same from fish to mammals, and the structure of the antidiuretic hormones displays only minor variations. The target organ for these hormones in mammals is the kidney and this in general is also true for the other vertebrates as well. There is the difference, however, in that in addition to the kidney the non-mammalian vertebrates have supplementary excretory organs, which act in combination with the kidney, and at times assume greater importance than the kidney, in the regulation of salt and water balance. Such a statement might have appeared startling a few years ago, but in the minds of comparative physiologists it is now well accepted.

All birds possess paired glands situated near the eyes, with ducts draining into the nasal cavity (Fig. 4.5). The glands produce a fluid which is eliminated

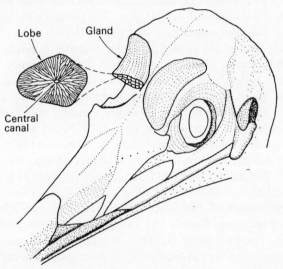

Figure 4.5. The salt gland of the gull consists of longitudinal lobes about 1 mm in diameter; each lobe has a central canal with the branching secretory tubules arranged radially around it. (Drawing by M. Cerame-Vivas.) (From K. Schmidt Nielson (1960) The salt-secreting gland of marine birds. *Circulation*, **21**, 962, by permission of the American Heart Association Inc.)

from the body via the external nares. Some birds eject the fluid by a characteristic side to side shaking of the head, but most allow it to run off the end of the beak; the petrel eliminates the secretion by a 'water pistol' mechanism using the expired air from the lungs to atomize the fluid contained in the nasal cavity and the tube on top of the beak.

Birds in their natural environments face dehydration by one or two causes, reflecting the main characteristic of their habitats. Marine birds face dehydration through excess salt, whilst terrestrial birds in hot climates or in situations where fresh water is at a premium face the same physiological stress through the unavoidable loss of water due to evaporative loss and the need to lose some water through the kidney in the excretion of waste metabolic products. The end result is the same, namely a rising concentration of salt in the internal environment of the animal.

Most of the work on salt glands in birds has been carried out on marine species and also experimentally on domestic birds such as ducks and geese which possess functional salt glands. The fluid which originates from the activated salt gland has been found to be essentially a NaCl solution which is more concentrated than sea water. Here then we have a mechanism whereby marine birds can avoid Na^+ accumulation and survive indefinitely on a diet containing sea water as the only source of drinking water. It is this mechanism that enables birds to live on oceanic islands and survive long transoceanic migrations without access to fresh water.

The conclusion that functional salt glands are found only in birds associated with marine environments has had to be modified since the observations that many terrestrial birds of desert habitat, including the ostrich (*Struthio camelus*), a North African partridge (*Ammoperdix heyi*) and several species of falcons have functional salt glands. It may be supposed therefore that the extra-renal route of electrolyte balance described originally for marine species may be of widespread importance in birds.

The interesting suggestion has been made recently that salt gland function is a prerequisite for birds to take full advantage of the water economy inherent in uric acid excretion. The argument runs as follows. Uric acid cannot be concentrated to a point where the kidney tubules become clogged. Therefore, the uric acid must arrive at the cloaca with a large amount of water. The watery admixture of faeces and urine is then regurgitated into the lower intestine where the bulk of the water is reabsorbed. This water is probably removed from the uric acid mixture by an active transport of Na^+ with a passive following of water, in accord with the accepted view that active transport of water is energetically improbable and yet to be convincingly demonstrated in any biological system (except possibly in insects). Having of necessity reclaimed the water by absorbing a hypertonic solution of NaCl the bird is presented with an unavoidable salt load and the salt glands then come into play. Implicit in this idea is that as a result of Na^+ and water movement across the cloacal/intestinal wall the body fluids become concentrated with respect to NaCl and the urine is hypotonic. But the need to compensate for kidney water loss is only one part of the overall problem of the bird. Added to this is the gain of appreciable quantities of salts in the diet and in warm climates the loss of large amounts of ion-free water by evaporation from their respiratory surfaces. Thus the salt glands represent the final common pathway of water conservation and salt excretion demanded of the organism, as a result of a number of separate but related physiological processes arising from environments in which free water is always at a premium. The alternative is that the bird must have ready access to sufficient amounts of ion-free water so that the kidney alone can cope with Na^+ excretion when evaporative water loss is no longer a problem. Such is rarely the case for essentially marine birds or birds living in the hostile conditions of the desert.

The control of the salt glands of birds has received a great deal of attention. There seems to be a dual control comprising both a neural and a hormonal

C

component. It seems clear that the initiation of secretion is via the para-sympathetic nervous system by the release of acetylcholine.

Also, it would seem that the endocrine system contributes to the maintenance of the internal environment at a number of levels within the organism which directly or indirectly affect nasal gland function. These levels can be generally described as tissue, systemic, and behavioural.

A direct action on the salt gland cells is suggested for corticosterone since an intracellular accumulation of this hormone in the active gland has been demonstrated. Prolactin and arginine vasotocin seem also to have a direct stimulatory action although the precise action of all these hormones remains in doubt.

Additionally, thyroid hormone might have a calorigenic role at the level of the salt gland and this hormone together with corticosterone might serve to maintain the availability of substrate (glucose) in the blood and therefore regulate its supply to the tissue of the salt gland. At the behavioural level it would seem that prolactin might be secreted in excess amounts to offset periods of isolation from free water such as occurs on nesting sites. It has been suggested that it might additionally serve to 'anticipate' periods of hypersalinity when adults and fledglings move from the dehydratory conditions of the nesting sites to the more saline conditions of the marine/estuarine feeding locations; in this sense the role of prolactin might be considered as a by-product of reproductive activities. Prolactin might in terms of daily activity be released in response to dehydration, and this hormone might induce the bird to increase its water intake although the value in terms of water gain relates of course to the salinity of the available water.

Environments such as the desert deny the animal ready access to water and dehydration is an important physiological hazard. It would seem that the vascular compartments are maintained at the expense of the intracellular compartment and the nasal gland further contributes to the constancy of the electrolyte content of the blood by excreting NaCl; readjustments to the total body composition can then occur when water becomes available. The role of hormones in these transitory adjustments are not known but it is possible that the circadian release of prolactin is important in this respect and A.V.T. might also play a role. The converse of the desert environment is, one might suppose, the cold wastes of the polar regions, which birds have successfully colonized. Here too dehydration is a serious result of environmental pressures for there is low availability for long periods of free water due to ice and the low temperatures result in excessive evaporative water loss; hence the overall effect of heat and cold might be similar and the solving of the problem in terms of salt and water balance might be the same.

In conclusion there are undoubted claims for the participation of a number of hormones in processes which in their sum determine the level of response of the nasal gland to conditions of hypersalinity or dehydration. The apparently diverse environmental factors so far studied share a final common pathway in terms of the hormonal factors operating on the nasal salt glands but it is likely that the initiation of secretion is via parasympathetic stimulation and with the possible exception of prolactin and A.V.T. hormones are supportive rather than initiative in their effect.

In view of their evolutionary relationships, it is not surprising that some reptiles have been found to have functional nasal glands. The Galapagos Lizard (*Amblyrhynchus cristatus*) is marine and lives on the shores of the Galapagos Islands, where it feeds on a diet of seaweed. It produces a salty fluid from its nasal glands, which is expelled from the nostrils as occasional clouds of water particles, reminiscent of a puff of smoke from a fiery dragon! Sea snakes (*Hydrophidae*) are truly marine, the more primitive members returning to land to lay their eggs while the more specialized bear living young and remain at sea throughout life. These snakes, which are reputed to be the most poisonous have been little investigated and it is not known whether the nasal glands are functional or not. The marine crocodile has been found far out to sea, but normally lives in estuarine swamps. It may well be that crocodile 'tears' are in fact, secretions from the nasal glands, and the tears of pain which turtles are said to produce when laying their eggs on land may likewise be secretions from the nasal glands. Preliminary investigations using hormones on turtles suggest that the mechanisms responsible for salt secretion are similar to those described for birds at least as far as corticosterone is concerned. Interestingly it has been suggested that in marine reptiles feeding on invertebrates known to be rich in K^+, that the excretion of this ion is via both the kidney and the salt glands. These reptiles drink sea water in order to provide a vehicle (water) for the elimination of K^+ through the kidney; Na^+ loading which inevitably follows the drinking of sea water is no problem because of the phenomenal excretory capacity of the salt glands for this ion. Investigation on terrestrial lizards has shown, however, that the salt glands are possibly much more versatile in that they can switch the balance of electrolytes in the secretion in favour of Na^+ or K^+ depending on the relative proportions of these ions in their diet.

Extrarenal organs of excretion in fishes and amphibians

Birds and reptiles are not the only animals possessing organs which at times may assume a greater importance than the kidneys in the regulation of salt and water balance. Fish living in sea water and fresh water have, respectively, problems of water conservation and elimination. In sea water, which is more concentrated than the body fluids, the problems of fish are similar to those of marine birds. In other words, marine teleosts require a mechanism to excrete the excess salt which diffuses into the body from the environment and, in addition, a mechanism to restrict water loss (which in fish takes place by osmosis through the body surfaces—usually the gills). Although the urine volume is small in seawater fish compared with freshwater species, the restriction of water loss is not sufficient to keep the animal in water balance (Fig. 4.6). Consequently, marine teleosts drink sea water to make up the deficit. In so doing they take in considerable amounts of salt which must be excreted. Evidence points to the gill as the site for the removal of excess salt, the mechanism being in the form of a 'sodium pump'.

For teleosts in fresh water, the converse situation applies, because now the body fluids are about thirty times more concentrated than the external environment. Water now enters the body by osmosis and is excreted by the kidneys. Just

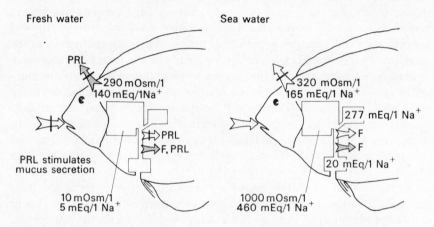

Figure 4.6. Hormonal control of water and sodium movement at the integument and intestine (boxes represent stomach, gall bladder and rectum). Open arrows represent water movement; cross-hatched arrows show sodium movement; inhibition is signified by a bar across the arrow; PRL (prolactin); F (cortisol). (From D. W. Johnson (1973) *American Zoologist*, **13**, 803.)

as in the mammal, the renal excretion of water also entails the unavoidable loss of salt. Some of the salt deficit is made up by the Na^+ in the diet, but an additional mechanism is required by freshwater fish to make up the Na^+ deficit and maintain a steady state balance. Once again the gills of the fish function to 'pump' Na^+, but this time from the external environment into the animal.

Some fish such as the salmon and the eel can live in both fresh water and sea water. What physiological changes take place in such migratory fish to enable them to move freely between the two environments? It would seem reasonable to conclude that some of the adjustments in, for example, the direction of Na^+ transport through the gills, are brought about by changes in the secretion of hormones. Debate still surrounds the question of the occurrence in fish of aldosterone, the mammalian salt regulating hormone, for it has been found only sporadically amongst the species so far examined. Cortisol is thought to play an important primary or possibly additional role in the regulation of both kidneys and gills (Fig. 4.7) and together with antidiuretic hormone appear to be involved in renal function in ways similar to those in which they aid survival of higher vertebrates. For example, the success of a salmon in migrating into fresh water may depend on its ability to switch from a seawater type of hormonal control, with high antidiuretic and perhaps low corticosteroid production, to the freshwater type of control with high corticosteroid and low antidiuretic hormone production, as the fish swims through the estuarine waters. This, of course, is an oversimplification, for the whole process of adaptation to the new environment

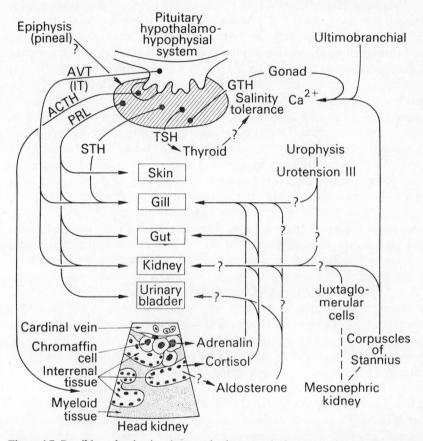

Figure 4.7. Possible endocrine involvement in the control of osmoregulatory effector organs. Apparent diversity of control may reflect imperfection or complexity of hydromineral regulation. (Adapted from D. W. Johnson (1973) *American Zoologist,* **13,** 800.)

seems to be very complex, and it is probable that hormones are only one of the factors concerned in the overall controlling mechanisms, which themselves are far from clear.

The posterior lobe of the pituitary in amphibians secretes a hormone which is antidiuretic in its effect on the kidney. This same substance has, in addition, the effect of increasing the absorption of water from the bladder and increasing the inward permeability of the skin to water. The concern of the antidiuretic hormone with a multiplicity of target organs has earned for it the title of 'water balance principle'. Amphibians are, with one recorded exception, either terrestrial or freshwater animals. Freshwater amphibians have the same problem as freshwater fish, in that there is a tendency for the animal to become flooded with water and to lose salt. Thus antidiuretic hormone would be expected to have little importance in such animals, but aldosterone plays an important role in promoting the active uptake of Na^+ from the environment through the skin, from bladder urine back into the body and through decreasing the loss of sodium through the kidneys. The antidiuretic hormone assumes real importance in the more terrestrial forms where there is a constant risk of dehydration. It acts by decreasing water loss and by accelerating recovery from dehydration when the animal returns to water. This hormone also enables the amphibian to draw on the water in its bladder which in frogs and toads is known to serve as an emergency water store. Of this phenomenon, Darwin in the *Voyage of the Beagle* wrote, 'I believe it is well ascertained that the bladder of the frog acts as a reservoir for the moisture necessary to its existence!' Other observers have frequently pointed out that some desert frogs (*Cyclorana*, *Chiroleptes*) store large amounts of dilute urine in the bladder when water is available after heavy rains. During prolonged periods of drought the frogs aestivate deep in the ground and slowly absorb the water in the bladder. The water reservoir is so large in these species that Australian aborigines, who perhaps live in one of the most hostile environments known to man, use the buried distended frogs as a supply of drinking water.

The observation of an amphibian living in sea water was not made until 1961, when the crab-eating frog (*Rana cancrivora*) was found in the sea off the coast of Thailand. The hormonal control of water and salt balance has not been investigated in this interesting species, but it is known that the problem of continuous dehydration found in marine bony fish is avoided in this frog by the retention of large amounts of urea in the body fluids, thus raising the osmotic pressure of the blood above that of sea water—a situation which closely parallels that found in the cartilaginous fish (the sharks and rays). In these fish, just as in the crab-eating frog, water diffuses into the body through the body surfaces because of the high osmotic pressure of the blood. Thus the drinking of sea water, which is necessary in the marine bony fish, is not required. By this unique method, cartilaginous fish and the crab-eating frog can remain in positive water balance. The cartilaginous fish display another interesting feature in the form of a digitiform gland situated in the fold of tissue which suspends the alimentary canal. This gland opens by a duct into the rectum, and it has been shown to be yet another 'salt gland', capable of producing a highly concentrated solution of NaCl at about twice the concentration found in the blood and higher than the concentration of NaCl in sea water. Thus sharks and rays have an extrarenal route of excretion of salt which, following either natural or experimentally administered salt loads, satisfies a physiological need of the animal in a manner not too dissimilar from that already described for the nasal glands of birds and reptiles and the gills of bony fish. The rectal gland of the shark, in common with the gill, responds to cortisol but whereas this hormone enhances excretion of Na^+ through the gill of the shark it blocks the excretion through the rectal gland.

In summary, it would appear that the hormones of the adrenal cortex and those of the posterior lobe of the pituitary gland are universally concerned in regulating the salt and water balance of the vertebrate body. These hormones appear to modify the properties of cell membranes in a way which secures an alteration in the rate at which salt and water pass between the cell and the bathing fluid in contact with the cell. The sites of hormone action are in specialized organs which, though they may differ greatly in gross appearance from one group of vertebrates to another, have in common the role of maintaining within carefully defined limits the salt composition of the blood and hence the content of the cell. Without such control salt concentration in the cells of the body would fluctuate widely according to environmental forces and these changes would eventually lead to death.

Gills and lungs

Specialized respiratory organs incorporate one or both of two main features; the general circulation is made to pass through a large number of tubes of small diameter which project into the external environment, and there is the anatomical provision whereby the external environment with which the blood exchanges, is replaced continually or periodically by a fresh supply.

Respiratory organs are classed as gills or lungs, according to whether the organ is composed of appendages projecting outside the body or into cavities within it. However, the distinction is not clear-cut because some animal species have aerial gills, whereas others have water-filled lungs. Two further common features are, that the volume of blood within the respiratory organ is large in relation to total blood volume and this in turn presents a large surface area for respiratory gas exchange with the environment and finally that the distance over which gases have to diffuse is short. Tracheal respiration found in insects, spiders and some other arthropods is unique in the sense that gaseous exchange with the tissues is effected by the direct contact of the cells with the gaseous environment via a complex of fine tubes called tracheae. These can be visualized as a fine network of tubes ending in the finest terminations called tracheoles where exchange occurs.

On the whole, lungs have the main role of taking up oxygen and removing carbon dioxide. In contrast, gills have important additional roles in the regulation of ion balance and in those aquatic animals that feed on suspended particulate matter, the gills provide also a system of filters which regulates the flow of particles into the alimentary tract.

Water currents necessary for the exchange functions of gills are produced in lower animals by the action of cilia, as in the lamellibranch molluscs, or by paddle-like appendages, as in some crustaceans. However, the most general method of ventilation involves the periodic expansion and contraction of the walls of the cavity in which the gills lie. It is also found commonly that these muscles are also involved in locomotion.

The gill system is most highly developed in the fishes. Water is drawn into the buccal cavity through the mouth and ejected over the gills through posterior gill slits. Muscles concerned with this lie in the wall of the buccal cavity, with the mouth and the flaps over the gill slits, acting as valves. A vital component in very active fish is the flow of water past the gills as the animal moves rapidly through the water. Air-breathing fishes which are often adapted to aquatic environments of low oxygen tension are able to fill the gill cavity with air when, of course, it ceases to function in the exchange of dissolved solutes.

With regard to true land vertebrates, air enters the lungs through the combination of special muscles associated with the ribs and diaphragm which expand the thorax. Expulsion of air results mainly from the inherent elasticity of the lungs and thorax. This process of ventilation is also a feature of organisms which do not possess real gills or lungs.

The hindgut is often modified to act as a water-filled lung, water being alternately drawn in and expelled again through the anus. Such a mechanism is found in some Annelids, insects and vertebrates, the air-breathing fishes and turtles.

The evolution of larger metazoans has necessitated the development of respiratory systems adequate to meet the demands of oxygen supply and carbon dioxide elimination. Circulatory systems help to eliminate the long diffusion pathways between the specialized areas for gas exchange at the body surface and the deeper lying tissues. The efficacy of the respiratory systems will depend to a large extent on the absorptive capacity of the circulating fluid for the respiratory gas. Thus the oxygen content of a fluid will vary according to the absorption coefficient (a measure of the absorptive capacity) and the partial pressure (pO_2) of oxygen. The pO_2 in the most favourable medium has a maximum value of about 160 mm and, therefore, the oxygen content of the blood can be augmented only by an increase in the absorptive coefficient. There are four coloured substances (respiratory pigments) which are used for just this purpose; haemoglobin, haemocyanin, chlorocruorin and haemerythrin. These respiratory pigments are different biochemically in the various phyla and even in the same phylum. The presence of one of these respiratory pigments increases the absorptive capacity of the fluids in which it is contained. These substances all show typical sigmoid absorptive or dissociation curves which describe how the amount of pigment combined with oxygen varies with the pO_2. The sigmoid nature of these dissociation curves (Fig. 4.8) serves to promote a large turnover of oxygen between arterial and venous tissues. In some animals, such as for example the squid (*Loligo*) the shape of the dissociation curve may be altered significantly by changes in pH such as those brought about by high concentrations of CO_2 in

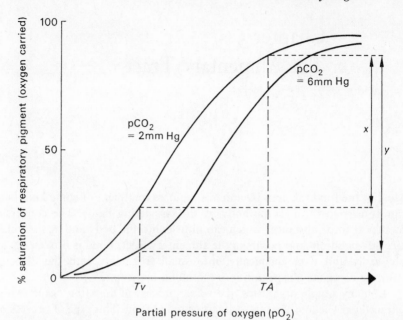

Figure 4.8. Hypothetical oxygen dissociation curve for a respiratory pigment showing a positive Bohr effect. *Tv*, *TA* = venous and arterial partial pressures of oxygen; *X* = total oxygen turnover if no Bohr effect was present; *Y* = total oxygen turnover between tissues when large Bohr effect is present. In some animals, such as *Loligo*, the extra turnover due to the Bohr effect may be as high as 30% but in mammals, such as man, it may be very small.

the body fluids. This phenomenon, the Bohr effect, operates in such a way that, since the pCO_2 in arterial and venous tissues will differ, the turnover of oxygen between these tissues is maximized. In some animals, such as for example the frog, juvenile stages have a dissociation curve shaped differently from that of the adult. In most mammals, the dissociation curves for foetal and maternal haemoglobin are displaced, so that haemoglobin in the uterine vein will give up oxygen to that in the umbilical vein.

Chapter 5
The Alimentary Tract

Most of the food taken in by animals requires treatment of some kind before it can be carried through the body by the circulating fluids. The conversion of foodstuffs into substances which can diffuse into the body and be assimilated is termed 'digestion' and occurs in the alimentary tract. Food is broken up, at first physically and then chemically, into small fragments with the objective of ensuring complete absorption into the blood or lymph.

In many simple organisms, the whole process of digestion occurs within an intracellular vacuole after the cell has engulfed food. This type of process occurs in coelenterates, platyhelminths and the lower molluscs alongside extracellular digestion, where food is dispersed mechanically in the alimentary canal and chemically disrupted by enzyme secretions.

A transitional stage between intracellular and extracellular digestion appears to be found in the coelenterates, where a central body cavity is present. Filamentous processes projecting from the inner walls of this cavity become wrapped around the particulate food; enzymes being secreted and digestive products absorbed locally at points of contact of filaments with the food material.

With regard to the more advanced invertebrates and vertebrates, the alimentary canal consists of a tube running more or less from one end of the animal to the other, with dilatations in various regions. These dilated sections may be closed off from neighbouring sections by means of rings of muscles, the sphincters, which control the passage of food from region to region. Functionally, there are three main parts: the foregut, the midgut and the hindgut. Starting in the region of the mouth, the foregut comprises the pharynx and oesophagous at its lower end. Organs with special functions may be developed, such as the crop, for temporary storage of food, the gizzard for mechanical disintegration and the stomach for mixing and enzymic digestion. The surfaces of the foregut do not usually secrete enzymes, but mucous secretions and enzymes may be added to the food by buccal glands in the mouth. In some animals, digestive enzymes are regurgitated from the midgut into the lower end of the foregut.

In terms of both form and function, the midgut is less variable, although in its two extreme types, it may be either a long convoluted tube or a dilated sac. Mucus and digestive juices are secreted into the lumen by the cells lining the tube or from glands which open into the lumen. Digestive diverticula are often found which may serve the purposes of digestion and absorption. On the whole, most of the valuable constituents of food are absorbed in this region.

The hindgut is a relatively simple and uniform structure, with the common functions of absorbing water and the preparation and expulsion of semi-solid waste matter.

It is not the purpose of this book to give an account of those processes of feeding and digestion which are adequately covered in standard texts. Rather the intestine will be viewed from the standpoint that it forms part of the boundary of the organism and, as such, interacts with its enclosed environment in a specialized manner, bearing in mind that this environment may be different in many ways from the environment of the whole animal.

Invertebrates

ORGANIC MATERIAL DERIVED FROM THE DIET

Many invertebrates rely partly, or almost entirely, on phagocytosis (intracellular digestion) for the final digestion and uptake of food material. In the higher invertebrates, with the exception of certain filter feeders, digestion is pre-dominantly extracellular. Outpushings of the intestine, digestive diverticula or caeca, are poorly developed in the annelids compared with the molluscs and arthropods but in the latter two groups they represent specialized areas for digestion and absorption. In the molluscs, and possibly the annelids, intra-cellular digestion is quite commonplace, particularly in filter feeding species. In the crustacea and insects, however, absorption takes place in the digestive diverticula or gastric caeca but not by phagocytosis. Indeed, in the insects the midgut is lined with a loosely fitting chitinous tube (produced either by the separation of thin sheets from the outer surface of the epithelial cells throughout the midgut, or secreted by a group of cells at the anterior limit of the midgut) which is called the peritrophic membrane. This appears to be primarily con-cerned with protecting the midgut epithelial cells from abrasion by food particles but is important in the present context in that it allows only soluble food material to enter the gastric caeca. Very little is known about the mechanism of absorption from the intestine in invertebrates in general but we do have some understanding of these mechanisms in insects.

The arthropod intestine is not a simple endodermal tube: while the midgut is of endodermal origin, the foregut and the hindgut arise embryologically from ectodermal inpushings and are therefore lined with cuticle continuous with that covering the body surface. This cuticular lining may be important in explaining some of the physiological properties of the insect rectum. Since the Malpighian tubes and rectum of insects form an excretory unit, these are discussed on pp. 44, 62 and 85–95 and the following account will be restricted to the insect midgut. In cockroaches and locusts the relatively short oesophagus is followed by a dilation of the foregut known as the crop (Fig. 5.1). Food in the crop is mixed with digestive secretions which have been passed forward from the midgut and with fluid from the salivary glands. It is in the crop that digestion takes place. With the possible exception of small quantities of lipid, no absorption occurs in the crop. Detailed experimental studies have shown that in the cockroach (*Periplaneta americana*) and the desert locust (*Schistocerca gregaria*)

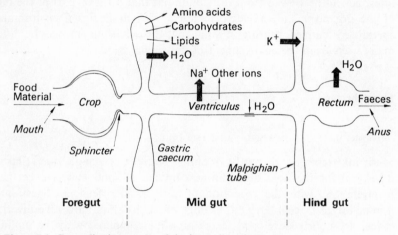

Figure 5.1. Generalized structure of the insect intestine.

triglycerides, sugars and amino acids are absorbed predominantly in the gastric caeca. Little or no absorption takes place in the remainder of the intestine.

Amino acids

Insects have a characteristically high concentration, probably higher than in any other animal group, of free amino acid in their haemolymph. The uptake of amino acids from the lumen of the gastric caeca must therefore present an appreciable problem. It must often take place against a considerable concentration gradient. When the intestine of *Schistocerca* is force-filled with an experimental solution isosmotic with the haemolymph, but which contains radioactively labelled amino acids and albumen, although labelled amino acids enter the haemolymph rapidly, the total amino acid concentration in the caeca increases to a level above that in the haemolymph. By following changes in the concentration of radioactively labelled albumen, which is not absorbed from the gut, it is possible to show that the volume of fluid in the caeca decreases to nearly half of its original volume after only 45 minutes! This suggests that water must be rapidly and preferentially absorbed from the caeca allowing amino acids to diffuse into the haemolymph along a concentration gradient.

Carbohydrates

Insect haemolymph, with a few notable exceptions, contains only small quantities of free monosaccharides. The principal blood carbohydrate is trehalose, a disaccharide of glucose, which is present in relatively large amounts. Glucose, and other monosaccharides, could therefore diffuse out of the lumen of the gastric caeca along a concentration gradient. This has been shown to be the case in both cockroaches and locusts. *In vitro*, diffusion of monosaccharides from the gut continues until the luminal fluid and the haemolymph are in equilibrium, but, *in vivo*, the absorption of sugars is facilitated by the rapid conversion of absorbed monosaccharides into trehalose. This conversion takes place in the fat body and the newly synthesized trehalose is released into the haemolymph. In this way the concentration gradient of monosaccharides across the gut wall is actively maintained. Uptake of water from the lumen of the caeca must also help in maintaining this gradient. Haemolymph trehalose may only leak back very slowly into the intestine since it appears that the intestinal epithelium, like other tissues of the insect, is relatively impermeable to this carbohydrate. Any trehalose which enters the gut lumen, either by leakage from the haemolymph, or more rarely, in the diet, is hydrolysed to glucose by the enzyme trehalase, produced by the intestinal epithelium. Glucose liberated in this way passes into the haemolymph, along a concentration gradient, in the normal manner. This facilitated diffusion of glucose is in direct contrast to the active transport of glucose across the gut wall in mammals.

The rate at which dietary material leaves the crop is clearly important. If the crop allows so much food material to enter the midgut that carbohydrate is diffusing across the gut wall faster than it can be converted into trehalose by the fat body, then the concentration gradient across the intestinal epithelium can no longer be maintained. Consequently, release of material from the crop is regulated so that the trehalose synthetase system is not saturated. The rate of crop emptying is known to be inversely proportional to the osmotic pressure of the crop fluid. The walls of the crop possess osmoreceptors which control, via the stomato-gastric nervous system, the action of the muscular sphincter between the crop and the midgut. This system of control over crop emptying is similar in principle to that in mammals but, in the rat for example, the rate of gastric emptying is not controlled by the total osmotic pressure of the stomach contents but appears to be specifically and directly related to the glucose concentration. In the insect, the response of the crop emptying mechanism to osmotic pressure means that the amino acids, sugars, fatty acids, other organic molecules, and inorganic material present in the diet, can all influence the rate of crop emptying by virtue of the osmotic pressure exerted by their solutions.

UPTAKE OF WATER AND INORGANIC IONS

Marine invertebrates are usually in osmotic equilibrium with their environment;

although they are known to show considerable regulation of their internal ionic composition. It is inevitable that part of the external environment will be taken into the intestine with the food. Since the intestinal wall must be relatively permeable to small molecules, to allow the uptake of dietary materials, it is likely that ions and water molecules pass across the intestinal wall fairly freely. In the majority of marine invertebrates this will present no osmotic problem and the ionic adjustments will be made by the appropriate organs. In freshwater invertebrates, however, which are faced with the possibility of continuous entry of water into the body fluids by osmosis, a large influx of water through the intestine would pose a considerable osmotic problem. It is known that freshwater invertebrates do not drink their environmental medium to any appreciable degree, but other mechanisms within the gut may also play a part in preventing osmotic flooding.

In the brine shrimp (*Artemia salina*) a crustacean which can survive and maintain its internal osmotic pressure within narrow limits, over great extremes of salinity (from 10% sea water to saturated brine), drinking of the external medium is of great importance. If a dye is introduced into the medium it enters the intestine from both ends and becomes appreciably concentrated in the midgut. Using phenol red, a dye which can be measured spectrophotometrically, it has been shown that the gut fluid is concentrated seven-fold by the time it reaches the midgut. An analysis of the midgut fluid shows that the osmotic pressure of fluid in the lumen is always greater than that of the haemolymph. However, in hypertonic media (25% sea water) the osmotic pressure of the gut fluid is markedly less than that of the external medium. It is thought that large amounts of Na^+ and Cl^- are actively transported from the gut lumen and water follows these ions passively. The greater osmotic pressure of the gut fluid over that of the haemolymph, therefore, is not due to sodium and chloride ions, but is probably caused by the increased concentration of bivalent ions such as Mg^{2+}, Ca^{2+} and SO_4^{2+}. Concentration of such ions takes place in marine teleosts which are also known to drink their medium. Large crystals are often found in the intestine of *Artemia* and while these have not been analysed chemically, it is likely that they consist of $CaSO_4$ crystallized out by the concentrating mechanism.

By swallowing its medium, therefore, *Artemia* is able to take in large volumes of water. The excess salt absorbed with this water is excreted by the first ten pairs of gills (p. 88). This water maintains the osmotic balance of the animal and prevents desiccation. Such a method of hypotonic regulation is also shown by marine teleosts (p. 58) where the drinking rate is thought to be determined by the osmolality of the medium. In *Artemia* acclimatized to 100% sea water, the drinking rate is about 2% of the body weight per hour but it is not known whether the drinking rate varies with the external salinity. Several marine palaemonids (prawns), which are thought to be freshwater-adapted forms that have returned to the sea, are known to swallow their medium and the gut may be as important in these forms, as a homeostatic organ, as it is in *Artemia*.

The larvae of the mosquito (*Aedes detritus*) which are adapted to live in water with a high salt content, are also known to swallow their medium. Excess salts taken up from the gut lumen are excreted via the Malpighian tubes (p. 45). It seems that the anal papillae, which in the freshwater form (*Aedes aegypti*) actively take up salts from the medium, and are much reduced in *Aedes detritus*, are unable to switch their function, as do the gills of teleosts, from that of ion uptake to salt excretion.

Experiments *in vitro*, utilizing preparations of insect guts, have thrown some light on the rate of movement of ions across the midgut epithelium. The isolated midgut of the silkworm (*Hyalophora cecropia*) has been shown to transport potassium from the haemolymph side into the lumen at a rate of 20 μequiv/cm^2 of gut/h. With both sides of the gut bathed in identical ringer solution, the potential difference across the midgut wall is approximately 100 mV and the lumen side is always positive. Changes in this potential difference *in vitro* are observed which appear to be related to developmental events, such as pupation, but are not affected *in vitro* by juvenile hormone analogues or α-ecdysone; their significance is obscure. While transport of K$^+$ across the gut wall is common in insects, a notable case being the Malpighian tubes, there is some reason to regard the magnitude of this rate of transport in the midgut of *Hyalophora* as being exceptional. The haemolymph of *Hyalophora* is unusual in that it has a high K$^+$/Na$^+$ ratio. *Hyalophora* is a phytophagous insect, the diet being K$^+$-rich, and these apparent anomalies may be reflections of a specialized diet. However, not all phytophagous insects have this high K$^+$/Na$^+$ ratio in their haemolymph.

In the cockroach (*Periplaneta*) the isolated ventriculus (Fig. 5.2) has a potential difference of 12 mV across the gut wall and the haemolymph side is positive. This is in direct contrast to the situation in *Hyalophora*, but is probably the more usual situation in the insect midgut. The potential difference across the gut wall in *Periplaneta* is sensitive to the action of metabolic inhibitors such as 2,4-dinitrophenol (DNP) and iodoacetamide. Ouabain, a cardiac glycoside which is believed to be a specific inhibitor of membrane ATPase and linked Na$^+$-K$^+$ pumps in a variety of invertebrate and vertebrate tissues, when placed on the haemolymph side of the gut wall, causes an irreversible loss of potential difference. When placed on the luminal side, however, it is ineffective; a situation reminiscent of its effects on the mammalian intestine. These observations suggest that the potential difference is actively maintained. Na$^+$ is the principal ion actively transported across the cockroach midgut epithelium. The use of radio-isotopes has shown that the balance of Na$^+$ efflux from the gut lumen, above the passive efflux measured in ouabain treated preparations, is of the order of 0·2–0·25 μequiv/h. This is a measure of the active transport of Na$^+$ from the gut lumen. The passive influx of Na$^+$ from the haemolymph side can also be measured. Making certain assumptions about the surface area of the gut it is possible to estimate the net efflux of Na$^+$ as being 4·83 μequiv/h/cm^2. This value agrees well with similar estimates for the rabbit intestine.

When the isolated ventriculus of *Periplaneta* is filled with a solution containing radioactively labelled inulin (to which the gut wall is impermeable) independent of the original concentration of the luminal fluid with respect to the bathing medium, the concentration of inulin remains constant. Therefore, although ions are removed from the gut lumen there is no net water movement. This finding is in direct contrast to the uptake of water from the gastric caeca. When DNP is present on both sides of the ventricular wall the net water movement follows that expected by osmosis. This suggests that some type of DNP-sensitive mechanism is normally present in the ventriculus, but not in the gastric

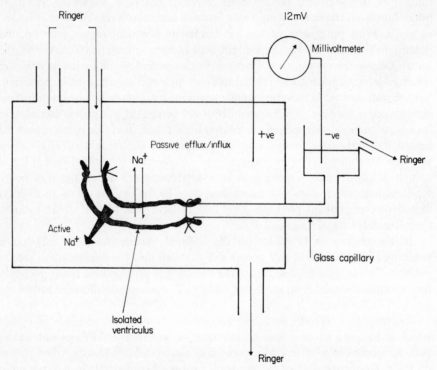

Figure 5.2. Measurement of transepithelial potential of isolated ventriculus.

caeca, which retards the passage of water across the ventricular wall. This restricting influence on water movement may be modified by the action of hormones, thus giving the midgut great potential as a homeostatic organ. The exact nature of the mechanisms involved are unknown but histological studies on the epithelial cells in the gastric caeca and the ventriculus have revealed that these cells, in common with other secretory cells and those of the Malpighian tubes and rectum, have an extensive system of basal infoldings. The possible physiological significance of such structural findings will be discussed in a later section.

Vertebrates

In general, the vertebrate alimentary canal functions in the same way as that of invertebrates, although we have more detailed information on special function for some of the more widely used experimental animals.

The intestinal epithelium is practically impermeable to polysaccharides. There is evidence that disaccharides may enter the gut cells and hydrolyse to monosaccharides. Many hexoses and pentoses pass through the walls passively. On the other hand, glucose and galactose are also transported actively by mechanisms, the nature of which is not fully understood.

By far the greatest amount of ingested protein is hydrolysed to amino acids before absorption. Although the dicarboxylic amino acids, glutamate and aspartate, appear to enter the body solely by diffusion, other amino acids enter by active transport; two mechanisms appear to exist: one for neutral compounds and the other for basic amino acids.

The question of lipid transport is open to debate. Regardless of the form in which fat is transferred from the lumen into the epithelial cells, it is present as triglyceride when it enters the lymphatic vessels. Experiments with radioactively-labelled triglyceride indicates also that between 25–60% of the hydrolysis occurs before absorption. Most of the remaining fat appears to be absorbed as monoglyceride.

Electron microscope studies suggest that fat may enter cells of the intestinal epithelium in microdroplet form by pinocytosis; a process of engulfment. However, diffusion of emulsified glycerides and fatty acids is more widely accepted as the basic mechanism of uptake. Water and monovalent electrolytes move readily through the intestinal epithelium. Water is transported passively, although its movement is usually coupled with the active transport of NaCl. The bulk of Na^+ appears to move into the body by active mechanisms, whilst most of the Cl^- ions move passively. Di- and trivalent ions do not readily enter the body, but where the ion constitutes an important item of the diet, such as Ca^{2+}, Fe^{2+} and Fe^{3+}, specific transport processes are found in the wall.

Other functions of the intestine

The intestine may take on many other functions, both as a receptor and as an effector organ, which are often, but not always, allied to its dietary function. The role of receptors in the insect crop, which influence the crop emptying rate, has already been discussed. Stretch receptors in the insect intestine may regulate not only feeding behaviour but also influence endocrine activity. In some insects, distension of the intestine due to feeding triggers off stretch receptors in the body wall and this initiates a whole series of developmental and physiological events such as moulting and egg production. The role of the intestine as a site for the production of chemical messengers or pheromones will be mentioned in a later section (pp. 168 and 180).

In some invertebrates the intestine may function as a respiratory organ. In the freshwater oligochaetes (annelids) water movement in and out of the rectum, by the action of the ciliated rectal epithelium, facilitates the exchange of respiratory gases across the gut wall. In the holothuroidea (echinoderms) more elaborate structures, the branched respiratory trees, are formed in the hind part of the intestine. Contractions of the posterior part of the alimentary canal drive water through these trees and their branches which terminate in thin-walled ampullae bathed in coelomic fluid. Respiratory gas exchange takes place across the walls of these ampullae. In some species the lower branches of the respiratory trees are modified to produce a sticky secretion which has a defensive function.

Part III
Specific Interactions of
Organisms with the Environment

Part III

Chapter 6
Global Diversity and
Animal Distribution

Life requires a constant supply of both energy and materials. There is only one important source of energy: atomic energy reaches Earth as light from the Sun. Every day, the surface of the Earth is bombarded with light equivalent to the energy of over a hundred million atomic bombs. Much of this energy warms the surface of the Earth and a further quantity causes the evaporation of surface water producing the air currents which transport the clouds of water vapour in fixed paths around the globe. Only a very small fraction of the Sun's energy is captured by life.

Sunlight is not distributed equally on the Earth's surface. Taking the Earth as a globe placed in the path of light which arrives in parallel rays at the equator, a given amount of light is spread over a larger area of the globe the nearer we are to the poles (Fig. 6.1). In these regions, we never see the Sun directly overhead

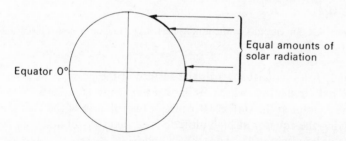

Figure 6.1. Distribution of radiant energy at low and high latitudes.

and light always hits the Earth at an angle, so that a large proportion is reflected off. Also, the Sun's rays have to pass through a greater amount of atmosphere, with the result that more light is scattered and therefore never reaches the ground. As a consequence it is not surprising to find that the Sun appears weaker at these latitudes and the Earth's temperatures are lower.

Only a small fraction of the radiant energy from the Sun is absorbed by the Earth's atmosphere. The remainder is either absorbed by the Earth's surface or is reflected back into space. Energy absorbed by the surface is re-emitted as heat.

However, this heat energy is not lost and a large fraction of it is taken up by the clouds of water vapour in the atmosphere. In this way, the moist atmosphere acts as a heat trap. Very little of the heat is lost to outer space and most is reflected back to the land and water surface. This principle of heat reflection is made use of by gardeners when they construct a greenhouse. Glass acts as the heat reflector in the same way as clouds. Indeed, the general phenomenon by which radiant heat from the Earth is conserved, is termed the 'greenhouse effect'.

The atmosphere is also heated from below by currents of rising hot air resulting from the Sun's action on land and sea. The overall result of direct and indirect heating is that the atmosphere is not heated equally. Radiant energy is more concentrated at the equator (Fig. 6.1) and the rising air is replaced by surface air from either side (Fig. 6.2). The rising air spills over north and south

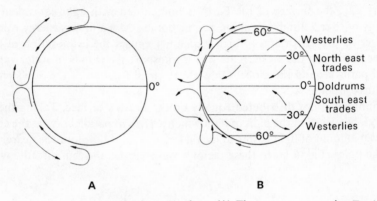

Figure 6.2. Air currents in the atmosphere. (A) Flow on a non-rotating Earth. (B) Actual flow.

and gradually loses its heat towards the surface at the poles. This gives rise to the meridional circulation, where air moves along the meridians of longitude towards the equator at the surface. Because of the rotation of the Earth, most of the air leaving the equator at high altitude is caused to cool and sink before it reaches the poles at about latitudes 30° N and S.

The complication produced by the rotating Earth can be understood by imagining a man standing close to the north pole. As the Earth rotates, he will move through space with a speed of rotation similar to that of the global surface at that point. During each twenty-four hours he will pass through a much smaller circle than a man standing on the equator. If the man on the equator could move due north very rapidly, he would move into an area where the Earth's spinning surface is relatively speaking moving less fast. He would, therefore, increase his speed relative to the Earth's rotation and would veer into the direction of rotation, i.e. to the east. By similar reasoning, an object moving due south would move to the right in the northern hemisphere and to the left in the southern hemisphere. The agency at work here is called the Coriolis force.

By the Coriolis force, the bulk of warm air from equatorial regions moves back to the equator and veers to the right and left in the northern and southern hemispheres, respectively, giving rise to the north-east and south-east 'trade' winds. The remaining 'equatorial' air carries on moving north and south beyond latitude 30°, drops at about latitude 50° and mixes horizontally with polar winds. 'Equatorial' air moving at these mid-latitudes veers into westerly winds, whilst the polar winds—moving towards the equator—veer easterly.

Air expands as it rises at the equator because it has less weight of air above it. It automatically becomes cooler and is then unable to hold moisture, just as warm air produces a film of moisture when it strikes a cold object such as a window-pane. The trade winds pick up water from the oceans and as they rise at the equator, deposit this as heavy rainfall in the Tropics. At about 30° N and S, the air falls, is warmed and picks up moisture resulting in a prevalence of deserts in these regions.

The prevailing trade winds cause surface currents in the oceans flowing west above and below the equator. When these currents reach the east shores of Asia and America, they are deflected towards higher latitudes to return along the west continental coasts. These two masses of circulating water in the Atlantic and Pacific oceans send heat to high latitudes in the 'west', with cold water moving to lower latitudes in the east. Where cold ocean currents occur off-shore on the western sides of continents, the associated blanket of cold surface air prevents the descending equatorial air from picking up moisture (cold air is heavier than warm air). These phenomena occur at about 30° N and S and tend to reinforce the desert aspect of the environment. When cold and warm air meet, fog is produced and this is often the principal source of moisture for plants in these regions. When surface water is moved by off-shore winds, it is then replaced by the 'upwelling' of deeper water which is often richer in mineral nutrients. The water currents running along western continental coasts also tend to veer away from shore, giving the same result. These off-shore upward moving currents of cold water often give regions of high biological productivity. Where westerly winds blow onto west coasts between 40–60° latitude off a warm ocean, there is a second zone of heavy rainfall.

If a bucket of sand and a bucket of water are placed together in the sun, the sand will heat up far faster and to a higher temperature than the water. It will also lose heat faster than the water. In the same way, during the day, land heats up faster than the sea, causing sea breezes to blow, whereas at night the air flow may be in the opposite direction.

On a much larger scale, the differences in the heating and cooling effects of land and sea, produce the asiatic monsoons. Great heat is absorbed during the summer in the interior of the continent, causing dry air to rise which is balanced by warm moist air from the Indian and Pacific oceans. This air brings sudden violent rain storms to the southern and eastern parts of the continent. During winter, the interior cools down to very low temperatures, reversing the air flow which blows as icy winds over a large peripheral area from the middle east to western Russia. The resulting climate, with large extremes in temperature, is termed a continental climate.

Where a land mass makes contact with water, the large heat capacity of water tends to minimize the seasonal fluctuation in land temperature. Winters tend to be milder and summers cool. In temperate latitudes, with westerly winds, the eastern coasts experience more seasonal extremes in temperature than the west coasts. On the other hand, if the flow of westerly winds is blocked by high mountain chains, as in Canada and the USA, the maritime influence does not extend far inland. Another effect of mountains is to force air upwards, causing it to expand and cool and thereby precipitating its moisture on the seaward slopes. On the lee side, as the air falls, it is warmed and picks up moisture. The land down-wind of a high mountain range is often desert due to this rainshadow effect.

While the daily rotation of the Earth produces dramatic effects on air currents, it also produces twenty-four hour periodicity in energy impact. This periodicity, coupled with the seasonal progression of the Sun relative to the Earth's surface, is responsible for many biological phenomena. As the Earth moves around the Sun every day, one half of the globe is illuminated. Because of the inclined axis of the Earth, the extreme latitudes experience great fluctuation in day length (Fig. 6.3). When the Sun is directly over 23°N on the summer solstice (mid-June), the north pole will be illuminated throughout an entire revolution of the Earth, and a part larger than half of any parallel northern latitude will be illuminated. This results in excess day's light in summer (Fig. 6.4) and by symmetry, there will be a corresponding excess of night at the same latitude south of the equator.

As the Sun's relative position moves north and south, the excess of day at one time in summer equals the excess of night at the same place at the corresponding time in winter. Every part of the globe receives the same total amount of daylight (six months) but, whereas the equator has twelve hours of daylight all year long, the poles receive their six months of daylight in one continuous stretch.

The temperature variation corresponding to these seasonal changes in light have marked effects on the distribution of living things. In the sea, there is little seasonal change in temperature and light is a limiting factor. The increased light in the spring results in a vast growth of microscopic plants. In smaller bodies of water, the summer sun results in a warm layer of less dense surface water which does not mix with deeper layers. By the activities of animals in the deep layers these may become devoid of oxygen, whereas the surface layers may be depleted of nutrients due to the activity of aquatic organisms both plant and animal. This results in a seasonal decline in productivity. Mixing of these two water masses takes place in temperate clime during the winter. The surface water cools and eventually the whole body of water may reach the same temperature when mixing may occur by wind action. With extremes of cold, the surface layers may

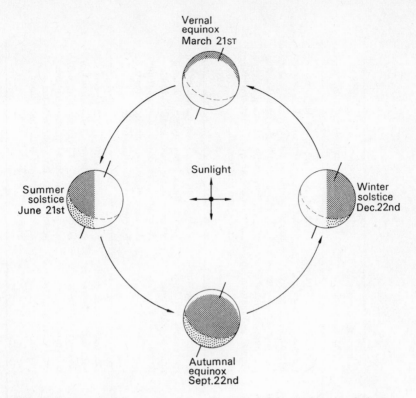

Figure 6.3. Seasonal differences in the sunlit portion of the northern hemisphere.

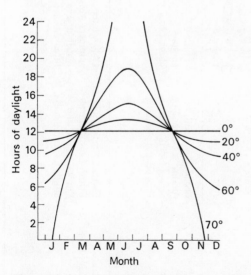

Figure 6.4. Annual changes in day length at different latitudes in the northern hemisphere.

Table 1. Biogeographical areas and their plant and animal associations.

Zone	Location	Main climatic features	Characteristic plants and adaptations	Characteristic animals and adaptations
Tundra	Northern zone encircling the Arctic Ocean.	Low mean temperature; long dark winters; short light summer. Frost likely all the year. Upper few feet of soil only thaws in summer and surface generally wet.	Shrubby alders, birches, willows and conifers. Moss cover extensive. Plants generally low growing with rapid growth and maturation.	Musk ox, reindeer, hares, lemming-like rodents, fox, polar bears. All well protected against cold by physiological and behavioural adaptations. Insects a common life form, with cold-resistant eggs and larvae. Numerous water-fowl breed during the summer.
Taiga	Broad zone south of tundra belt extending across North America, Europe and Asia.	Similar to tundra, but summer longer and climate less extreme.	Similar to tundra, but more trees with large areas of coniferous forest.	Mammalian fauna more varied than in tundra. Black bears, wolves, martens, lynxes and numerous small rodents. Adaptations similar to those of tundra dwellers. Numerous invertebrates which become dormant in winter.
Temperate deciduous forest.	Eastern North America, British Isles, Central Europe, China and South-Eastern Siberia.	Cold winters, warm summers with well-distributed rainfall and little seasonal variation.	Deciduous trees dominant with wide species diversity. Common ones are beech, sycamore, oak, elm and poplar.	Browsing deer, wild pigs, large cats such as puma, panther, etc. (all varieties of Felix concolor). A high percentage of species are arboreal, particularly tree-nesting birds. Invertebrate fauna associated mainly with forest floor habitat.

Rain forest	Central America, Northern South America, Central Africa, Southern Asia, East Indies, South Pacific Islands and parts of N.E. Australia.	High rainfall, humidity and temperature with little seasonal variation in day length.	Very wide range of tree species, and forest a characteristic mixed community dominated by climbing vines and epiphytes. Vertical stratification of plant forms well marked.	Ground-dwelling herbivores, e.g. musk deer, small antelope, pigs and rodents. Arboreal species well represented, e.g. leopard, jaguar, snakes, monkeys. Numerous bird species, many with poor powers of flight. Frogs particularly well represented. All groups of invertebrates represented in large numbers.
Grasslands	N. America east of the Rocky Mountains, Venezuela, East Africa.	Low intermittent rainfall, unevenly distributed.	Many grass species adapted to special conditions of soil, rainfall and evaporation.	Dominated by large herbivores adapted to conditions of open country. Rodents very common. In general, small mammals are burrowing or fossorial. Predators include wild dogs, lions, etc. adapted to herbivorous prey. Many kinds of herbivorous invertebrates such as locusts. Insect-eating birds common and many herbivorous species.
Deserts	S.W. U.S.A., Western South America, Arabia, North Africa, Western China and Mongolia, Central Australia.	Low rainfall and intense sunlight. Nights generally cold and evaporation rate high.	Annual plants common with rapid growth rate. Perennial plants are succulent with leaves reduced or absent. Characterized by long root systems.	Large mammals scarce. Numerous small rodents adapted to the scarcity of water and extremes of temperature. Snakes and lizards very common.

actually become colder than the bulk of the water in this situation. The surface waters, being heavier, sink and mixing thus takes place.

Another important aspect of seasonal temperature difference is that in many parts of the world, rains are seasonal. Rainfall in winter produces a larger proportion of water available for plant growth than rainfall in summer, simply due to the higher rate of loss by surface evaporation in summer.

Set against the great range of physical diversity of the Earth, we can see that the distribution of any species of organism is limited by the distribution of suitable environments (Table 1). We know that communities differ with latitude and living things have their own characteristic geography. However, the present-day physical conditions do not provide the whole explanation for the geography of organisms, and many aspects of plant and animal distribution are due to differences in the history of the regions. Organisms came to them at different times and from diverse places and evolved independently once they were there.

Temperature, solar radiation and rainfall are the major factors that control plant communities. In one way or another, all animals are linked to plant communities and the conditions which determine the existence of plant communities also control that of their animal dependants. On the other hand, zoologists have only, to a limited extent, been able to define animal communities comparable with the major botanical divisions because of the powers of locomotion and physiological and behavioural adaptability which enable animals to evade direct environmental control. Nevertheless, each of the main biogeographical regions of the Earth has one or more special morphological and physiological characteristics that enable the fauna to cope with the major physical conditions of the environment.

Chapter 7
Adaptations to Specific
Environmental Problems

With regard to terrestrial regions, we may define six major climatic zones. The tundra, taiga and alpine communities, the temperate deciduous forests, the rain forests and deserts. The geographical location, major habitat features and animal adaptations are set out in Table 1 (p. 80).

Clearly the ranges of environmental variables encountered by animals are very wide. Air temperatures range from −70°C in the polar regions in winter to above 45°C, which is a characteristic shade temperature in the Sahara desert in summer. Water temperatures range from the freezing-point of sea water, about −2°C to above 40° in hot springs. Light conditions vary widely from total darkness in deep caves to a brilliant glaring light found on white coral sand in the Tropics. There is also a wide range of atmospheric pressures from sea level at about 1 atmosphere to less than a half of this value on the 5,000 metre peaks of the Andes and Himalaya; hydrostatic pressures differ more profoundly, from 1 atmosphere just below the sea surface to 1,000 atmospheres at the bottom of marine trenches in the Pacific Ocean. Salt concentrations range from zero in the melt water from inland glaciers to nearly three times as concentrated as sea water in enclosed marine bays and inland lakes subject to intense solar radiation. To all of these variables must be added the geographical variation in the detailed chemical composition of the soil and terrestrial waters; wind velocity, day length, oxygen concentration of natural waters and the recent changes brought about by man's activities. It is the adaptation of animals to these different conditions that have resulted in present-day diversity of form and function.

On the whole, the physiological capabilities of animals in the temperate zones are not of great ecological importance in the determination of their distributional limits. It is more likely that the distribution is limited by other factors such as competition, predation, food supply or availability of suitable physical habitats. On the other hand, in many areas of the world, the physical environment is very demanding and severely limits the fauna. Some of the most demanding environments are found in the low latitude deserts which occupy large areas of continents and oceanic islands on both sides of the equator and extend north and south on the lee sides of mountain ranges, particularly in North and South America.

In these extreme habitats, we find a limited range of animals but in all areas of the world, there is an almost infinite series of physical situations available and animals can, by their behavioural adaptations, select the most suitable environment in a very precise way that allows their anatomical and physiological attributes to function adequately for survival and reproduction.

Heat and cold

For convenience, animals are classed as homeotherms and poikilotherms, the former group regulating body temperature whereas temperature of the latter group varies with the temperature of the environment. Neither group is independent of changes in environmental temperature. Energy must be expended by homeotherms to maintain body temperature different from that of the external environment, the energy expenditure being proportional to the temperature differential. On the other hand, in poikilotherms, since body temperature is not regulated except through behaviour, energy expenditure varies directly with the environmental temperature.

The few species found in deserts also exhibit certain features common to other animals living in areas such as the Arctic, where physical conditions are the main limiting factor. The two major features to which desert animals must adapt are high temperatures and water scarcity, coupled with the existence of large changes —both daily and seasonally—in temperature and rainfall.

Adjustment to these extreme conditions are varied and numerous. Complete avoidance of severe heat load takes place by special nocturnal and fossorial behaviour patterns. Part of the heat load may be assimilated through physiological tolerance and the acceptance of a cycle of hyperthermia. Cyclic changes in body temperature may be of short duration, as in ground squirrels and antelopes which are very active for brief periods of time followed by quiescent periods when their behaviour is designed to dissipate the heat accumulated. In contrast, the camel shows a steady diurnal activity pattern and it has adapted to tolerate a correspondingly slow rise and fall in body temperature throughout the twenty-four hour period.

Behavioural control of heat exchange is a common pattern in reptiles, which maintain a steady body temperature by moving along a temperature gradient according to the relative ratio of heat loss and gain. Some lizards have mechanisms to regulate their rates of heating and cooling, so extending the periods of time that can be spent at or near this preferred temperature.

Birds, in general, exploit sustained hyperthermia as a device for facilitating heat loss, and it appears that some desert birds can also reduce the metabolic rate as a way of minimizing heat load. Birds show also mechanisms for heat dissipation that involve a minimum of energy expenditure and/or a minimum of water loss. In this respect, the webbed feet of young birds may serve as effective heat dissipators, as do the readily flattened gular areas. Heat exchangers are found widely in poorly insulated appendages and serve to cool the appendage without reduction in blood flow. Conservation of heat also takes place in appendages; both heat exchange and conservation take place through a special anatomical feature where vascular bundles of many arteries are arranged in parallel with thin-walled veins surrounding single arteries. All of these systems are countercurrent arrangements in which heat from warm arterial blood is exchanged to returning venous blood before it reaches the surface of the appendage.

In some animals, there is a shunt, whereby the heat exchange can be by-passed for the rapid dissipation of excess heat during exercise. Heat exchangers are found in tail flukes of porpoises, the feet of penguins and wading birds and rabbit and elephant ears. However, it must be stressed that tissues of many homeotherms exposed to marked temperature fluctuations often show the property of maintaining normal function at temperatures that might be considered lethal. Examples of this phenomenon are found in the peripheral tissues of cold-acclimatized rodents (cell division) and birds (nervous conduction).

The simplest adaptation to heat load is quiescence which occurs widely in desert birds and mammals. This may be extended to a condition of torpor at certain critical periods of the day. The problems encountered by animals living in polar regions are also primarily those of regulation of body temperature.

The limitation of the activities of animals can be eased by compensatory adaptive processes requiring several weeks or months for completion. For example, in fishes, cold acclimatization occurs by a gradual elevation of metabolic rate, so that a greater level of activity is possible. Homeotherms adapt by two principal means. Insulative changes result in extension of the zone of thermoneutrality to a low temperature, together with a reduced rise in heat production below the critical temperature. Metabolic adaptations give an increased capacity to maintain high rates of heat production. Partial relaxation or abandonment of temperature regulation is also practised in many species as an adaptation to cold, termed 'torpor' or 'hibernation'.

Homeothermy greatly extends the thermal limits for survival and activity. In poikilotherms, little adaptation is possible to temperatures below freezing. Fishes exposed to cold may show lowered lethal limits of between 5 and 10°C, and certain species may live when supercooled to $-1\cdot7°$ in sea water. Arctic mammals, in contrast, may be active indefinitely at below $-40°$.

Availability of salts and water

INVERTEBRATES

Considerable numbers of sea-living invertebrates and nearly all endo-parasitic animals live in isosmotic environments and thus may be thought to have little or no osmotic or ionic problems. However, it must be remembered that although organisms may indeed be isosmotic to their environment, their particular ionic content may be very different from that of the environment. Animal cells contain many organic anions not found in the external medium, such as, for example, amino acids, lactate, acetate. Moreover certain ions such as K^+ may be at a much higher concentration within the animal than in the external medium. Thus, as outlined in Chapter 2, an essential prerequisite for osmotic and ionic regulation is that animals possess semi-permeable membranes and ion pumps either selectively to remove ions from cells or to take ions up into them.

The problems of electrolyte balance have existed since the organization of the first cell. This organization occurred in sea water and thus it is likely that problems of water balance were not of prime importance in the early stages of evolution. When animals are in a steady state of equilibrium with their normal environment (that is the environment characteristic to that particular species) they maintain their water and ionic contents at relatively stable levels. The maintenance of a steady state is possible because of the osmotic adjustments made to the body fluids by specialized tissues. The majority of marine invertebrates are in osmotic equilibrium with their environment. However, many groups have evolved from marine ancestors to invade fresh water and land by various routes; through estuaries, up the shore or through the brackish water of swamps. There has been a subsequent reinvasion of the sea and its shore by such groups as the marine pulmonate molluscs; moreover brackish and sea waters have also been invaded by the terrestrial insects. It is only in this radiation of organisms from the sea that water balance became a problem and it is in these successive new environments that animals meet with special problems of osmotic and ionic regulation. Special osmotic stress also occurs when organisms take on an aerial existence and are faced with an increased risk of desiccation (see also pp. 55–56).

In conditions of changing salinity many organisms are unable to prevent the concentration of their body fluids altering passively towards that of the external environment—such animals are said to be osmoconformers. Animals which are able to maintain their body fluids at a more or less constant concentration irrespective of the concentration of the external environment are osmoregulators or euryhaline animals. Some animals are able to tolerate only rather limited changes in the concentration of their external medium and these are known as stenohaline animals.

Some osmoconformers can survive and indeed live comfortably over a large range of osmotic concentrations. The flat worm (*Procerodes*) lives in estuaries and is periodically exposed to fresh water. During osmotic flooding it has been shown that the animal increases considerably in size. Provided there is a small amount of calcium in the external medium an equilibrium is reached and the animal is able to exclude or remove some of the excess water. However, large amounts of the water which enter osmotically pass through the tissues and are stored in vesicles in the endoderm (gut lining). Contrary to expectation these vesicles are not discharged into the gut, but when the animal returns to sea water the vesicles shrink and the flatworm decreases in volume. The fact that fluid is segregated implies a precise control of water balance at the cellular level. The way in which the concentration of the body fluids of two annelid worms change in relation to changes in the external environment is shown in Fig. 7.1. Both *Nereis pelagica* and *Arenicola* are osmoconformers and the concentration of the body fluids is exactly in step with that of the external medium. However, another annelid (*N. diversicolor*) shows a marked ability to osmoregulate and maintain its blood concentration above that of the external medium. The shore crab (*Carcinus*) in contrast to *N. diversicolor* begins to osmoregulate immediately the

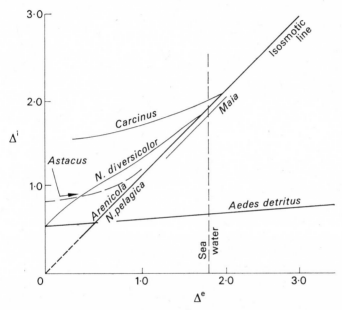

Figure 7.1. The relationship between the concentration (expressed as the depression in freezing point △) of the internal medium with that of the external medium for a number of invertebrates. For details see text. Sea water freezes at – 1·87°C. (Based on Scheiper (1929), Beadle (1939) and Ramsay (1952).)

sea water begins to become diluted. The nereid worm tolerates a much greater drop in the osmotic pressure of its blood before commencing to osmoregulate.

Other marine crabs such as *Maia* are stenohaline and only able to survive in a very narrow range of salinities (Fig. 7.1). Freshwater crustacea such as the crayfish (*Astacus*) may tolerate also only a narrow range of salinities but in this instance the range is of dilute solutions (Fig. 7.1). Other animals exemplified by the brine shrimp or the larvae of the mosquito (*Aedes detritus*) can tolerate a very wide range of salinities from almost distilled water through to very brackish water (Fig. 7.1). In *Artemia* both the gut and gills are involved in ionic regulation. This small animal (a large adult weighs only 8 mg) can survive in a surprisingly wide range of salinities. It will survive in crystallizing brine and is

D

regularly found in salinities some 10-fold greater than that of sea water or down to as little as 10% sea water. Moreover, in laboratory conditions it can survive in distilled water for 24 hours. It survives in this range of habitats by constantly drinking the water which surrounds it. The water along with the NaCl is absorbed through the gut epithelium, the excess salts are then actively excreted through the gills present on its first 10 pairs of legs. This mode of survival in an hyperosmotic environment is of course very similar to the way in which marine teleosts survive in their hyperosmotic environment (p. 57). The water taken in during drinking of course restores that which is continually lost to its hyperosmotic environment.

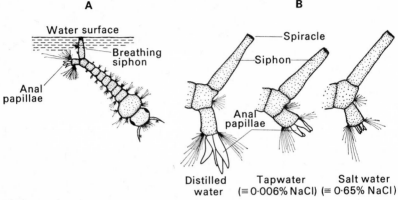

Figure 7.2. (A) To show the position of the anal papillae in a larvae of the mosquito, *Culex pipiens*. (B) Posterior end of larval *C. pipiens* reared in different environments, showing the different sizes of the anal papillae. (From V. B. Wigglesworth (1965) *Principles of Insect Physiology*. Methuen & Co. Ltd.).

The larva of the fly *Ephydra cinerea* is able to survive in the salt lakes of Utah, which have a salinity equivalent to a solution of 20% NaCl. The blood of the larva has a rather high osmotic pressure, which alters very little whether the larva is in distilled water or 20% NaCl solution.

The larvae of mosquitoes are aquatic; the gut and the anal papillae (thin circular flaps) are concerned with osmoregulation but in quite a different way from the brine shrimp. For example in the larvae *Culex* the anal papillae are freely permeable to water and salts. The water entering the insect is continually removed *via* the Malpighian tubes (p. 44). The Cl⁻ content of larvae reared in distilled water is reduced to a level equivalent to 0·05% NaCl and when the larvae are subsequently transferred to tap water (in which the chloride content is still low, i.e. less than 0·006% NaCl) the larvae are able to take up Cl⁻ through their anal papillae. Indeed the uptake of Cl⁻ is so effective, that even in this environment, the larvae can readily restore the Cl⁻ content of the blood to its normal level of approximately 0·3% NaCl. The size to which the anal papillae grow depends upon the salinity of the environment. In Fig. 7.2. it can be seen that the anal papillae are larger in those larvae from dilute solutions. The increased surface area presumably facilitates the uptake of ions. The absorptive cells of the anal papillae are rather similar in structure to those of the Malpighian tubes (Fig. 7.3 and compare with Fig. 4.2). Anal papillae cells have extensive infoldings of both the apical and basement membranes, with associated mitochondria. The active uptake of Na^+ and Cl^- may be achieved by independent mechanisms but the processes are most efficient when both ions are being

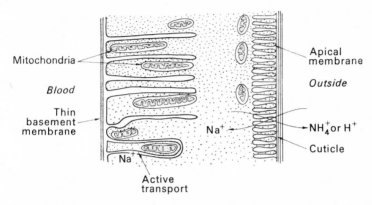

Figure 7.3. Diagram of an anal papilla cell of a larval mosquito. See text for details of functioning.

transported. Na^+ uptake is achieved by exchanging external sodium for hydrogen or ammonium ions and external Cl^- is exchanged for hydroxyl or bicarbonate ions. The active ion pumps for Na^+ uptake may be present at the basal membranes whereas the sites of ion exchange for Cl^- uptake may be present on the apical membranes (Fig. 7.3).

In the majority of aquatic and terrestrial invertebrates the excretory organs play an important role in osmoregulation. For example, aquatic crabs, like many other seawater organisms, have blood levels of Mg^{2+} and SO_4^{2-} which are much lower than the levels in the surrounding sea water. These low blood levels are maintained not by passive processes but by the action of the antennary gland (Fig. 7.4). If the Mg^{2+} concentration of the external medium is increased there is no associated increase in blood levels, but the concentration of Mg^{2+} in the urine is increased markedly. This increase in urinary Mg^{2+} concentration could be brought about in a number of ways. However, measurement of the rate of clearance of inulin from the blood shows that at least half of the urine originally formed is absorbed during its passage along the urinary tube. Since the urine voided from the crab is isosmotic to the blood some ions in addition to fluid must also be absorbed from the urine. These selective reabsorptive processes bring about the concentration of unwanted substances in the urine. Indeed even in intertidal forms or those crabs which spend a considerable time on land, and in which it would be most beneficial to restrict water loss by producing an hypertonic urine, the urine produced is isosmotic to the blood. The capacity of enzymatic processes and other essential mechanisms to function efficiently when the

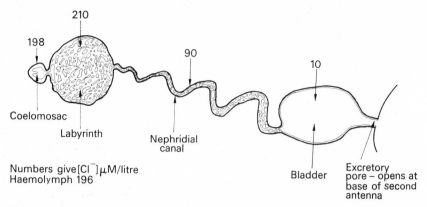

Figure 7.4. Diagram of an 'unravelled' antennary gland of the crayfish, *Astacus*. In this group of arthropods the excretory tubule is supplied with arteries which provide the hydrostatic pressure necessary for filtration into the coelomosac. The chloride concentration, obtained by micropuncture studies, is a rough indication of salt concentration. The salt concentration in the ultrafiltrate present in the coelomosac is the same as in the haemolymph, which indicates the probable filtration of all ions into this sac. Reabsorption of salts then occurs along the length of the excretory tubule most likely by active processes. This filtration-reabsorption process enables the crayfish to produce a markedly hypotonic urine.

internal osmotic pressure falls, together with the waterproofing of the integument, and the active uptake of ions by the gills constitutes collectively the major adaptation to hypotonic environments. With the exception of *Astacus* the crustacean kidney assumes little importance in osmotic regulation.

TERRESTRIAL INVERTEBRATES

Of all the terrestrial arthropods, the terrestrial crustacea are perhaps least fitted for life on land both in relation to their waterproofing mechanisms (p. 35) and the functioning of their excretory systems. So far we have only mentioned terrestrial or semi-terrestrial crabs but of course there are crustacea such as woodlice which spend all of their life on land. But again these animals have inefficient waterproofing and lose large quantities of water in their urine. They survive because of their habit of living under stones, debris, etc. where the microclimate can be surprisingly humid. Woodlice and other terrestrial crustacea retain the vestiges of their aquatic ancestry in that they still excrete their waste nitrogenous material as NH_3. This of course necessitates the production of a dilute urine. The other better adapted terrestrial arthropods restrict their water loss in the urine by producing insoluble nitrogenous wastes, such as uric acid (in insects) and guanine (in spiders). In general the only concession shown by woodlice to restricting water loss in the urine is to show a general reduction in nitrogen metabolism and thus reduce the amounts of NH_3 produced.

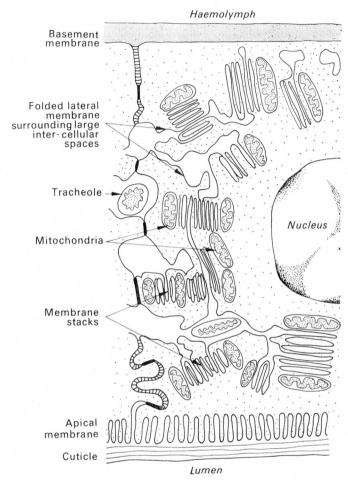

Figure 7.5. Diagram of the more important ultrastructural features of a rectal papilla cell. The large intercellular spaces communicate with the flattened stacks of inter-cellular membrane. These membrane stacks possess an active ATPase and are probably the site of active ion transport. The stacks are sandwiched between mito-chondria. It is important to note that the basal membrane which is bathed in haemo-lymph is much reduced in surface area compared with the apical membrane facing the lumen of the rectum. (From M. J. Berridge (1970) in *Insect Ultrastructure*, Ed. A. C. Neville. Blackwell Scientific Publications Ltd.)

In woodlice the rectal glands may absorb some water from the faeces, but they are especially important in enabling the animals to replace their body water by taking water up through the anus and absorbing it into the blood through the rectal pads. Thus woodlice drink not only through their mouths but also through their anus.

In terrestrial insects and also in aquatic ones the rectal glands are important organs in osmoregulation. As well as absorbing water from the urine the glands are able to absorb Na^+, K^+, and Cl^- against concentration gradients of up to 100-fold and probably all by active processes. Most of this information comes

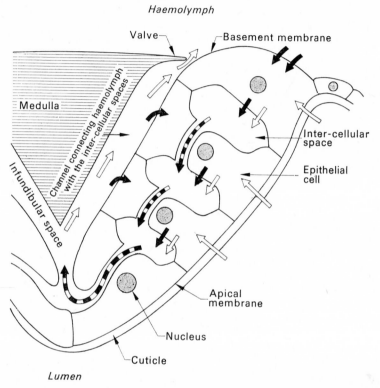

Figure 7.6. Schematic longitudinal view of an insect rectal papilla showing the route of fluid movement from the rectal lumen to the haemolymph. The large intercellular spaces connect, through a valve, with the haemolymph. Illustrated is the uptake of water (open arrows) across the papilla into the haemolymph in the absence of net uptake of solute. Solute (closed arrows) is recycled by being returned into the rectal pads across the basement membrane or solute may be recruited from the haemolymph. This recycling of solute means that water is dragged into the epithelial cells from the lumen. (From M. J. Berridge (1970) in *Insect Ultrastructure*, Ed. A. C. Neville. Blackwell Scientific Publications Ltd.)

from studies on the desert locust. In this insect the cuticular lining covering the rectal glands has water-filled pores which are 70Å in diameter. The cuticle is 10–100-fold more permeable to water than to KCl or NaCl and larger molecules such as disaccharides can only penetrate the cuticular lining slowly. Thus the cuticular sieve restricts the movement of large molecules, but water, salts and amino acids pass through very readily. There is still of course the possibility of further selection in the compounds reabsorbed by the action of the rectal glands themselves. Not only are a number of ions, salts, sugars and amino acids re-absorbed through the rectal epithelium into the blood, but the epithelium and rectal glands are capable of concentrating the urine to a marked degree. Indeed some insects can produce faecal pellets which scarcely contain any water at all. This movement of water back into the blood through the rectal wall can take place against an osmotic gradient and, moreover, this movement of water can take place independently of the transport of any ions or other solutes. These cellular mechanisms are still speculative, but recent detailed ultrastructural studies of the rectum have enabled a plausible hypothesis to be formulated. It seems likely that ions are actively transported into the intercellular spaces; the major site of active ion transport being the infolded lateral membrane stacks. These stacks (Fig. 7.5) are sandwiched between mitochondria and are rich in ATPase. Thus the stacks are readily supplied with the energy necessary for the functioning of the ion pumps. This active movement of ions creates osmotic gradients along which water moves passively. As more water enters the intra-cellular spaces a hydrostatic pressure will develop which forces water into the infundibular space. Ultimately the pressure generated will be sufficiently large to force water through the valve, into the haemolymph.

The movement of water from the lumen into the haemolymph is thus depen-dent upon the generation of very high localized concentrations of ions and other solutes within the intercellular spaces. Ions can be recruited either from the lumen or recycled from the infundibular space or haemolymph. This recycling of ions explains of course why water movement from the lumen can occur in the presence and absence of net uptake of solute (Fig. 7.6).

URINE VOLUME

The concentration of ions and metabolites in the urine is important in osmo-regulation but the absolute amount of urine produced must also be taken into account. Obviously if the volume of urine produced is large the loss of ions in the urine can be large, even if the ions are at a relatively low concentration. In the crab (*Pachygraspus*) which lives on the sea-shore the volume of urine pro-duced is 15-fold greater in 50% sea water than in normal sea water. In crusta-ceans as in the majority of other invertebrates there is only a passive regulation of urine volume. However, in a number of insects this is not so and although particularly well adapted to conserving body water, the control of water content is complex. It is essential for some insects, especially those which suck plant or animal fluids, to dispose of the very large amounts of water taken in with their food. The blood-sucking bug (*Rhodnius*) takes large meals and within some 2–3 hours of feeding may have produced its own weight in urine. The majority of aquatic insects produce continually a copious urine which removes not only the water taken in during feeding but more importantly also removes that water which enters the body by osmosis. Many other insects face temporarily the problems of excessive intake of water. For example, the herbivorous desert locust needs to eat its own weight in food each day to provide sufficient raw materials for growth and reproduction. On a diet of fresh grass or lettuce this results in a daily intake of 1,500–2,000 μl of water each day. The blood volume of the locust is only some 500 μl and thus it is imperative that the excess water be removed. However, when water is at a premium due either to cessation of feeding (perhaps for as little as a few days or in the case of blood-sucking bugs for many weeks) or when aquatic insects are placed in an hyperosmotic environment, the volume of urine produced is markedly reduced. During periods of starvation the urine voided by *Rhodnius* is a semi-dry sticky mass, quite unlike the clear watery urine voided after feeding. Likewise, in an hyperosmotic environment the Malpighian tubes of mosquito larvae fill up with solid matter and little or no urine is passed from the insect. Thus the volume of urine is controlled to a fine degree and water is only lost in the urine or faeces when excessive amounts have been taken into the body.

The regulation of urine volume has been shown to be controlled by hormones in a number of insects. In *Rhodnius* the effects of extracts of various tissues on preparations of isolated Malpighian tubes has shown that a diuretic hormone is produced by neurosecretory cells which are present in the posterior part of the thoracic nerve ganglion. If the ventral nerve cord is sectioned, the release of hormone, which occurs after feeding, is prevented. Thus release is occasioned by the extensive stretching of the abdomen which occurs at feeding. Messages are relayed from the abdominal stretch receptors *via* the ventral nerve cord to the thoracic ganglion and these signals bring about the release of hormone into the blood.

In the desert locust the diuretic hormone is produced by the brain neurosecretory cells and stored in the corpora cardiaca (p. 143). The action of the hormone is to increase the rate of excretion through the Malpighian tubes but additionally this hormone restricts the reabsorption of water from the rectal lumen through the rectal wall into the blood. The overall effect is to increase the amount of water lost through the excretory system. Feeding is one of the primary factors which brings about the release of the diuretic hormone in the locust and this of course is very similar to the situation in *Rhodnius*. This is obviously an effective self-regulatory mechanism; the process which leads to an increased intake of water into the body is also responsible for switching on those systems necessary to eliminate from the animal any possible excess.

During periods of water conservation, locusts release an anti-diuretic hormone from the glandular lobe of the corpus cardiacum. This hormone does not affect the Malpighian tubes, but does markedly increase the rate of reabsorption of water through the rectal wall. Thus water balance can be maintained or body water content increased by the action of such an anti-diuretic hormone, without restricting excretion through the Malpighian tubes.

In the locust, excretion and rectal reabsorption are regulated by a fine balance between hormones acting antagonistically. In *Rhodnius* the blood of non-feeding individuals contains no diuretic hormone and the presence or absence of this hormone from the blood may allow a sufficient fine control of the excretory system in such an intermittent feeder.

CHANGES THROUGHOUT THE LIFE HISTORY

The osmotic and ionic problems of some vertebrates but of very many invertebrates can of course change markedly throughout their life history and it is incorrect to think of all developmental stages of a species being solely adapted to live in only one type of environment. For example, in those insects with a pupal stage, the larvae can be very dissimilar in form and have a very different mode of existence from the adult stage. For example, mosquitoes have terrestrial blood-sucking adults and aquatic larvae which feed upon detritus in the water. However, even organisms in which the body form may not exhibit such marked changes during development may still show considerable variety in the environments in which the different stages live. Perhaps this is best exemplified by a group such as the parasitic nematodes. All stages of these organisms are essentially aquatic but the tonicity of the environment of the various stages differs markedly. The free living larval stages are primarily soil dwelling and thus like all other soil dwelling organisms have to cope with a constantly changing environment. The pores between soil particles generally contain air, but the particles themselves are covered with a thin film of moisture with larger pockets of water at their interfaces. When it rains, water surges through the particles overcoming the surface tension of the pores and the nematode larvae or other soil-dwelling organisms are quickly immersed in a very dilute solution. When the rain or flooding stops, the soil drains and water is drawn out of the pores by capillarity. Moisture is further extracted from the soil by evaporation and by uptake into plant roots. These processes of course increase the osmotic pressure of the soil moisture and can exert considerable stress upon the soil organisms. Thus soil-living nematodes are constantly being subjected to changes in the osmotic pressure of their environment. In the animal parasitic forms, the larvae adapt to changes in soil moisture and also have to cope with considerable drying when they are exposed on the surfaces of plants or on the soil surface, before penetration or being eaten by the host. Once within the host both plant and animal parasitic nematodes have only to tolerate the same range of osmotic pressures as the host tissues.

VERTEBRATES

According to habitat, vertebrate animals encounter great differences in the availability of salts and water (Fig. 7.7) as great as those already described for invertebrates. This may either lead to adaptations designed to allow the organism to cope with certain well-defined conditions or to adaptations which enable the organism to live in environments that differ markedly with respect to daily or seasonal cycles. A detailed account has been given in a previous chapter (p. 43) of the mechanisms of osmotic and ionic regulation in vertebrates.

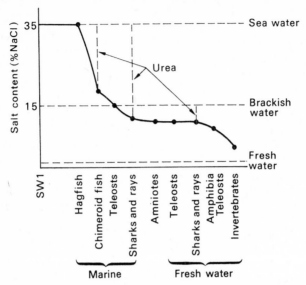

Figure 7.7. Osmotic pressures of body fluids in relation to the environment with particular reference to the urea concentration.

Pressure

BAROMETRIC PRESSURE

The gravitational influence of the earth upon its gaseous environment produces the phenomenon of barometric pressure. Since the gravitational field decreases exponentially with the distance from the Earth's centre, so will the barometric pressure. At sea-level, a terrestrial animal experiences a maximum barometric pressure of 760 mm of mercury. This atmospheric pressure will only change appreciably if the animal descends into a deep cave, for example, or ascends by climbing considerably above sea level; man may, of course, ascend by mechanical means to greater altitudes than are accessible to other animals. Such changes in barometric pressure are, however, of no great physiological significance in themselves. The major physiological problems of high altitudes are due to the problems of anoxia and low temperature rather than the reduced barometric pressure. Nevertheless, rapid ascent to high altitudes or rapid decompression can result in serious physical or mechanical injury or even death. It is calculated that a man decompressed suddenly to a pressure equivalent to that at 70,000 ft above sea level, would lose 1·8 litres of water by evaporative loss from the lungs before dying in about 3 minutes.

Many animals, such as, for example, some insects and spiders live permanently at altitudes much in excess of 18,000 ft (the highest permanent human habitations) while many birds undertake non-stop flights over mountain ranges. Little is known of the physiological adaptations shown by such animals to high altitudes but man shows marked acclimatization to the anoxia associated with high altitudes and this is concerned mainly with an improved efficiency of ventilation of the lungs and supply of oxygen to the tissues. A major feature of this acclimatization process is a marked tachycardia (rapid heart beat) which is in marked contrast to the adaptations in aquatic diving animals discussed in the following section.

HYDROSTATIC PRESSURE

An aquatic animal must withstand additional hydrostatic pressure to that of the atmospheric pressure prevailing at sea level. This hydrostatic pressure is due to the weight of water and it increases by about 1 atm for every 10 m in depth. Many air-breathing animals are specialized in such a way that they can endure submersion in water for long periods during diving. The major physiological adaptations shown by such diving animals are bradycardia (slow heart beat), the restriction of the circulation to the most essential areas and an insensitivity of the respiratory centre to lowered pH levels caused by higher levels of CO_2 and lactic acid during anoxia. Hydrostatic pressure, however, places a severe limitation on the depth to which most animals may dive.

The problems faced by man during deep-sea diving are well known. At great depths, unless some mechanical device is used to deliver air to the lungs at pressures equal to the hydrostatic pressure at that depth, the lungs will collapse. Such devices, however, create two serious hazards. First, under higher pressures, increased quantities of gases dissolve in the body fluids and these may reach toxic levels. Second, if the diver ascends too rapidly, these gases come out of solution and may form bubbles within the blood vessels (the diver experiences the 'bends') or the lungs may expand too rapidly and blood capillaries may rupture. Many diving mammals have overcome these problems by the possession of cartilaginous supporting rings in the bronchi which extend further into the lung than they do in terrestrial mammals. In addition, muscular sphincters prevent air flowing out of the alveoli and back into the bronchi when the air volume is decreased under pressure. Therefore the lungs are prevented from collapse and it is likely that the capillary circulation is reduced so that excessive quantities of gases are not dissolved during deep diving.

It has been mentioned above that hydrostatic pressure increased markedly with depth. Nevertheless, life exists in the deepest marine trenches where pressures may exceed 1,000 atm. Laboratory experiments have shown that such pressures may produce molecular rearrangements in proteins. Physiological adaptations to pressure in truly barophilic organisms have not been studied since there are great technical problems in collecting and studying such animals under normal conditions.

Many marine animals, especially planktonic forms which undergo diurnal vertical migrations, respond to changes in hydrostatic pressure. Increase in pressure elicits usually an increase in swimming movements whereas decreases in pressure have the opposite effect. These changes in swimming activity in response to pressure changes are non-directional in the absence of further stimuli such as, for example, light or gravity.

An interesting example of an animal which responds to increases in hydrostatic pressure by less active swimming (and *vice versa*) is the amphipod, *Caprella*. This 'reversed' response to pressure changes may have a distinct selective advantage in littoral species since it would decrease the chances of the animal becoming stranded at low tide. The sense organs involved and the mechanisms by which *Caprella* and other crustacea detect pressure changes is unknown. It has been suggested, however, that electrophysiological mechanisms may respond directly to pressure changes since electrical models may be constructed which show pressure sensitivity.

BUOYANCY

There are two theoretical mechanisms by which animals may adjust their weight in order to counteract gravity (and become buoyant). They may exclude heavier elements or include lighter materials which may be incorporated into floats or buoyancy tanks.

Sea water has a specific gravity of 1·02, whereas that of protoplasm lies between 1·02 and 1·10. It has been calculated that a hypothetical invertebrate which contained body fluids isosmotic with sea water could obtain a lift of 26 mg/ml of fluid if its salts were replaced by fresh water. Clearly, this is an impossible situation in a biological sense, but a degree of hypotonicity could confer some buoyancy. In the luminescent protozoan (*Noctiluca miliaris*) it has been suggested that a degree of buoyancy is achieved by the partial replacement of NaCl with NH_4Cl. In a wide range of invertebrates it has been shown that buoyancy is achieved largely by the exclusion of SO_4^{2-}. For example, in many jellyfish, pteropod molluscs, and tunicates the body fluids are isosmotic with sea water, but are all of lower specific gravity by virtue of the partial exclusion of SO_4^{2-}. Many bathypelagic fishes have taken the drastic step of reducing their body protein content markedly by a reduction in the caudal and trunk musculature (swimming muscles) thus achieving a marked reduction in their total specific gravity. A most elegant and sophisticated technique for achieving buoyancy is found in the cuttlebone of the cuttlefish (*Sepia officinalis*). The volume of the fluid contained in this 'buoyancy tank' can be regulated by the osmotic movement of water in and out of the cuttlebone due to the activity of ion pumps in the vascular epithelium which covers its posterior-ventral surface. Since the cuttlebone is built of layers of calcified chitin it can withstand considerable pressures and the movement of water can vary its specific gravity from about 0·5 (containing about 10% water) to almost 0·7 (30% water). This allows

Sepia to swim to depths at which the hydrostatic pressure may exceed 20 atm.

Other animals achieve buoyancy by including lighter materials in their body thus; many large vertebrates such as whales and sharks store generous quantities of lipids. Indeed, many protozoa possess oil droplets which add to their buoyancy. The sharks contain relatively large amounts of the fatty hydrocarbon squalene, which has a specific gravity of 0·86; considerably lower than the corresponding figure of 0·93 for cod liver oil. Another cephalopod mollusc the deep sea squid (*Cranchia scabra*) has a large coelomic cavity (about 65% of the total body cavity) which contains about 480 mM NH_4^+ and only 90 mM Na^+. (In contrast *Sepia*, for example, has 465 mM Na^+ in its body fluids.) This accumulation of low density liquid allows the squid to achieve neutral buoyancy.

The buoyancy tank of *Cranchia* is bulky but it can be used at great hydrostatic pressures due to the virtual incompressibility of water. A further possibility of the inclusion of light materials to achieve buoyancy is to provide gas-filled spaces which can act as flotation chambers. Many floating plants and animals such as, for example, giant kelp, jellyfish, *Nautilus*, and some teleosts employ such gas bladders.

The gas chambers of fish (swim bladders) enable fish such as the cod and perch to achieve neutral buoyancy. The swim bladder occupies about 5% of the total volume of the fish and provides a lift which just balances the weight in sea water of the other tissues. It functions in two ways. First, small changes in depth are compensated for by expansion or contraction of the gas within the bladder and these changes alter the animal's buoyancy. Long term changes result in either a secretion of more gas into the bladder or a reabsorption of the gas back into the blood stream—and in this way neutral buoyancy is again achieved. The swim bladder is used down to astonishing depths possibly as far as 4500 m where the pressure will be around 450 atmospheres.

The proportion of O_2 in the gas increases with depth and in fish living at appreciable depths the gas is almost pure O_2. Thus it is clear that the swim bladder is capable of concentrating O_2 against steep pressure gradients. This capacity resides in the gas gland on the surface of the bladder. The secretion is intimately connected with a specialized structure called the rete mirabile which can be described simply as a network of arterioles directed towards the gas gland which break up into capillaries, which are in close juxtaposition with a similar network of capillaries returning blood from the gas gland. This counter current system allows a build up of a large gas pressure difference between the blood in the gas gland and the general circulation.

Excretion of waste nitrogen

Ammonia is a common waste product arising from the metabolism of a wide range of nitrogenous compounds and the form in which it is excreted varies in relation to the environment.

Free ammonia is toxic, even in very small concentrations, and many adaptations have evolved in order to prevent its accumulation in the body fluids. There are three main ways of excretion, namely rapid removal in solution, conversion to a more complex, but innocuous, material and the excretion of various complex metabolites of nitrogenous compounds before they are degraded to ammonia.

Ammonia is excreted, as such, only when there is an abundance of water for its rapid removal. With regard to animals in which water is at a premium, i.e. those living in terrestrial habitats and marine vertebrates that face constant osmotic desiccation, nitrogenous waste is excreted in a more complex form.

The terms ammonotelic (ammonia excretion), ureotelic (urea excretion) and uricotelic (uric acid excretion) describe the form of nitrogenous excretion in different animals. However these categories are not so clear-cut as was once thought (Table 2) since amino acids make up a significant proportion of the

Table 2. Main nitrogenous excretory product.

Animal group	Ammonia	Urea	Uric acid	Amino acids
Vertebrata				
Mammalia	x	xxx		
Aves	x		xxx	
Reptila				
Alligator	xxx	x	xx	
Turtle	x	xxx	xx	x
Lizards			xxx	
Amphibia	xx	xxx		
Pisces	xxx	x		
Selechia		xxx		x
Arthropoda				
Insecta	x		xxx	
Crustacea	xxx			x
Mollusca				
Cephalopoda	xxx			x
Gastropoda	xx	xxx		x
Bivalves	xxx			xx
Annelida	xxx	xx		x
Echinodermata	xx	x		xx
Protozoa	xxx			

KEY
  x   small but significant
 xx   common product
xxx   major product

waste nitrogen in some invertebrates, and the nitrogenous substances creatine, creatinine and trimethylamine oxide have been found in the urine of many animals. Creatine phosphate plays an important role as an immediate energy store in the muscles of vertebrates. Urinary creatine may partly represent an excess of this substance in the diet, but most of the excess is excreted as the anhydride creatinine. Trimethylamine oxide occurs especially in the urine of elasmobranchs and marine teleosts, where it may make up 25% of the excreted nitrogen. It has been shown that much of the urinary trimethylamine oxide comes from the invertebrates in the diet, and its role as an end product of ammonia metabolism is questionable.

In terrestrial animals all three categories of nitrogenous excretion are found. The main determinant is again the availability of water. This, of course, may vary during development. Some animals develop during a semi-aquatic existence, where the young are incubated in water or moist places, others in a viviparous condition where the embryo is, in fact, virtually aquatic, and a third category includes animals that develop in the closed egg or cleidoic environment, where the embryo is surrounded by an impermeable shell which encloses an aqueous habitat of relatively small volume. These conditions determine the main excretory product. In general, ammonia predominates in the waste products of the aquatic invertebrates. Urea synthesis was probably an emergency device for the first semi-aquatic forms, and uricotelism is regarded as the ultimate adaptation to a situation in which no water can be spared for dissolving waste nitrogen.

The excretion of different nitrogenous compounds provides an interesting example of biochemical evolution and is illustrated well in the ontogenetic changes described for the chick embryo. Here in the course of fifteen days the embryo passes through successive stages of ammonia, urea and uric acid production.

Chapter 8
Animal Rhythms

The scope of research

There is probably no definition of the terms 'life' and 'living' that would be completely acceptable to all biologists. The closer one examines living organisms, the more difficult it becomes to obtain a satisfactory all-inclusive definition of the life process. This difficulty arises because organisms are united at many levels; subordinate systems become integrated successively into cells, organs and organ systems. It is only at the level of the whole organism that one is on safe ground in propounding an all-embracing definition which enumerates the most important phenomenological characteristics of life. This Chapter deals with two of these characteristics which must impress all who study animals: first, the apparent directiveness of functions, as if the end state were 'desired' and fixed by some external agency responsible for steering the life process towards a goal; and second, the obvious fact that animal life is of a cyclical or oscillatory nature. There is a link between these two phenomena in that, at the chemical level of organization, oscillations in function appear to occur in anticipation of new needs. It is at this level that rhythmical activities are linked with changes in the environment.

Detailed study of any living system shows that its activity is not constant. There exist phases of high activity followed by phases of low activity. Certain of these variations alternate so regularly that it is possible to speak of rhythmical variations. Many of them are familiar to us: the alternation of waking and sleeping, the periodicity of menstruation in women and the seasonal flowering of plants.

Why does our heart need to beat? Why do we need to sleep at regular intervals? In what way are the mating seasons of animals determined? What is it that controls the regular or periodic flowering of plants?

There are only two basic ways of providing the answers to these questions. The first way is to say that the rhythmical movements of the heart ensure that blood, containing vital nutrients, is supplied to all the cells of the organism; we sleep to repair the wear and tear of our tissues. These answers are concerned with the functions of rhythms and are not, properly speaking, explanations of the phenomena.

The other type of reply is based upon an approach described as determinism. Spring is the mating season for certain animals because with the longer days, there is an increased stimulation of the sensory organs, then of the brain, then of the hypothalamus and pituitary whose hormones increase the activity of the gonads.

This second kind of answer is comprehensive and links environmental processes with physiological events; but the reply is never complete, because it is necessary to specify in detail how the brain excites the hypothalamus, how the secreted hormones act, and to translate these facts into terms of physics and chemistry. In these latter two fields of science, functional replies are not the usual method of approaching problems.

Looked at in this way, the field of biological rhythms is essentially an interdisciplinary one, in that questions, of necessity, arise at a very complex level of organization and the ultimate explanation comes from many complementary areas of specialization.

Elementary rhythms

The next section is an attempt to describe some selected examples of rhythmical activity which are manifest at an elementary level. This approach is taken on the assumption that from an examination of these basic activities, the lowest common denominators of rhythms may emerge.

The first example deals with the rhythm in respiration. This rhythm is only one example of several motor activities which are repeated with a characteristic interval. In man, some fifteen times a minute, a group of muscles comes into play to increase the thoracic volume and allow air to enter the lungs. This type of rhythm exists throughout the animal kingdom; in fish, for example, a group of muscles rhythmically modifies the buccal and branchial cavities so that water surrounding the respiratory tissues is renewed at regular intervals. These various muscles are not physiologically different from other skeletal muscles. If their motor nerves are cut, they become paralysed and respiration ceases. There is, however, a central nervous system control located in a restricted area of the brain. Destruction of this site leads to death from asphyxia. This respiratory centre is autonomous in that if it is isolated from the brain, spinal cord and peripheral nerves, rhythmical excitation of the respiratory muscles persists. How is the rhythmical activity of this small group of nerve cells maintained?

All experiments in this area have been carried out with the assumption that nervous rhythms are produced in response to cyclic changes in the concentration of blood components that are specifically dependent upon the process of breathing.

Famous studies in this area were carried out by Frederique who succeeded in supplying the head and trunk of the same dog with different bloods. Irrigation of the head with venous blood, with ample oxygen in air entering the lungs, resulted in a rapid respiration rhythm characteristic of asphyxia. Conversely, if the centre received arterial blood, respiration rate remained normal, even when the inspired air was abnormally high in CO_2. The present view is that nerves in the respiratory centre are activated by carbon dioxide and inhibited by oxygen, and that the rhythm largely depends on the balance between these two substances in the blood (Fig. 8.1).

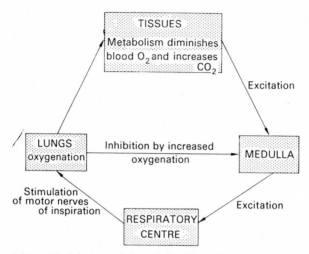

Figure 8.1. Diagram of the relationship between respiratory rate and blood composition.

The second example comes from work on the cardiac cycle. A heart separated from the organism will beat regularly for hours or even days, provided it is irrigated by a medium of appropriate composition and kept at a suitable temperature. Such an isolated heart appears to possess everything necessary for autonomous function.

In the most highly evolved animals the heart possesses generally two types of functional muscular tissue. The bulk of the heart is made up of muscle fibres joined together to form a network, the cardiac muscle. The other essential component is also contractile but present in small discrete areas termed *nodal* tissues. There is still much disagreement as to the relative importance of these two tissues. We know that both components are capable of rhythmical activity and that the degree of dominance depends on species.

The nerves to the heart play only a small part in the genesis of the heart beat. Some hearts are capable of automatic rhythmical functioning when they contain no nervous tissue. For instance, hearts of bird embryos beat before nerve cells make their appearance during ontogeny. Also, in molluscan hearts, there is no trace of nervous tissue, yet any part of the snail's heart no matter from which region it is taken will contract rhythmically when placed in suitable conditions.

Although the vertebrate adult heart contains a highly differentiated system of nervous and muscular origin, the nodal tissue is assigned the key role in the genesis of rhythmical contractions. One of the principal masses of nodal tissue is sited at the point of entry of venous blood; this is the sinus node. It has long been known that cardiac contraction in the frog and mammals begins in this region and is propagated to the auricles and ventricles. Also, in the failing heart, rhythmical contractions persist longest in the sinus. If the heart is divided, the parts distant from the sinus either cease to beat or beat with a much slower rhythm, whereas those connected to the sinus beat with the rhythm of the sinus.

In terms of its physiological significance, nodal tissue is an autonomous mass of cardiac muscle fibres that also have some of the morphological features of nerves. The main evidence for their role in conduction is the presence of large amounts of connective tissue between the fibres which could act as insulation.

The rhythmical activity of excitable systems is a mode of normal activity. When a sense organ is stimulated, a succession of electrical waves passes along the sensory nerve which are far from being aperiodic. Some isolated nerves, for example those of crustacea, are capable of rhythmical activity when exposed to the effect of a constant electric current, to desiccation or various unbalanced salt solutions. By modifying one or more factors in the solution bathing the nerve, it is possible to vary the amplitude frequency and period of the rhythm. From experiments of this type, it can be concluded that rhythmical activity is autonomous and that the characteristics of the rhythm depend on various environmental factors. Some natural factors also initiate rhythms, for example, muscular rhythms are started by traction resulting from the filling of the heart with blood or the gut with food.

In looking for an explanation for rhythms in excitable tissues, early workers thought that the refractory period might be responsible. During one part of systole, the heart is refractory to all stimuli reaching it. When we try to excite a nerve at a point where a nerve impulse is passing along it, the new stimulus is ineffective. For an excitable tissue submitted to a constant stimulus, the nature of the refractory period means that after the initial response, the tissue behaves as if the stimulus had been interrupted. This interpretation appears to account for a number of rhythmical phenomena but is not generally valid because in many tissues, the period of the rhythm is shorter than the refractory period.

Basic spontaneous rhythms are usually of short duration. The higher frequency rhythms are found at autonomous nervous transmission and muscular contraction (maximally at about 2,000 c/sec). Neural rhythms are either concerned with the generation of impulses in single neurons (1–1,000 c/sec) or constitute oscillatory systems built of several neurons and sometimes including muscle with frequencies from about 20 c/sec to durations measured in hours. Related phenomena are the limits for our perception of rhythms (5–50 c/sec) or rhythms in our mental activity (0·3–80 c/sec). Rhythmic muscular activity occurs involving striated muscle (walking, chewing, tapping, breathing 0·3–8·0 c/sec) and non-striated muscle (vascular tonus, peristalsis 10 sec–several days). These are controlled by nervous tissue.

True myogenic rhythms exist in heart and insect flight muscle: the latter contracting at a higher rate than that of the nerve impulse (35–2,200 c/sec).

Possible maximum oscillatory rates may be calculated from the rate of discharge of neurons (1–1,000 c/sec), synoptic delay (0·5–1·0 msec), length of nerve fibres and conduction velocity (1–10 msec) as well as from data on non-neural components, such as length of muscle fibres. In general, cortical systems (with small distances between neurons and without non-neural components) should oscillate more rapidly than local motor feedback systems; and the latter should perform faster than motor functions regulated by feedback through long nerve trunks. Actually the electroencephalogram contains components faster than the 7 c/sec of the motor system.

Furthermore, small animals should show oscillations that are more rapid than larger ones, having shorter neuron paths, smaller mechanical mechanisms, etc. Actually, there is, in a double log plot, an inverse linear relationship between the heart rate or respiratory rate and body size. Heart rate in mammals ranges between 1,000 beats/min in dwarf bats (4 g body weight) to 20 beats/min in the elephant (2,000 kg body weight). The upper limit is about 17 c/sec.

In non-striated musculature several superimposed classes of rhythms seem to be created by autonomous control centres. Blood pressure shows rapid variations with durations of 10, 20, 60 secs and 2–15 minutes. Heart beat includes variations in rate of 15, 30 and 60 secs superimposed on the basic rate.

Definitions

The importance of periodicity in living phenomena has never been underestimated but it is only recently that it has been studied scientifically and systematically.

A fundamental concept is that of the *duration* or *period* of the cycle. In this discussion we are only concerned with processes for which the time interval separating two identical physiological, morphological or biochemical states may be considered constant. This eliminates all those phenomena classed as cyclic but shown to be aperiodic, for example, certain parasitic 'cycles'.

Although most biologists acknowledge that an adequate terminology and satisfactory definitions are indispensable, no international agreement has been reached. Rhythm, cycle and period are used interchangeably to designate the regular variations of a biological process.

It has been proposed to reserve the word *cycle* for intrinsic variations: in other words, for those actually belonging to the biological system considered. The word *rhythm* would then designate variations of *extrinsic* origin, i.e. those imposed upon the biological system by regular modifications of the environment. This proposition gives rise to difficulties in that it seems that most of the known biological rhythms and cycles are not intrinsic.

Other workers make use of the phrase 'physiological clock'. This expression highlights the intrinsic characteristics of the process but the word clock also evokes the undesirable image of a particular type of mechanism.

Research on biological rhythms has concentrated to a great extent on those with a period of about 24 hours. Such rhythms have been classified as diurnal rhythms or daily rhythms. These designations are misleading because they include both the phase corresponding to the light period (the strict definition of diurnal) and the diurnal and nocturnal phases together. The use of the expression, 24-hour rhythm does not take account of the fact that most rhythms do not last exactly 24 hours, but 24 hours plus or minus a few minutes or a few hours.

In the face of this confusion many workers have adopted the convention proposed by Franz Halberg and use the term *circadian* to describe these short-term rhythms. It is formed by the junction of two Latin roots, circa (about) and diem (day). As a new term with no language overtones it appears to be the best way of designating this type of cyclic variation. The corresponding term for periods longer than 24 hours, for instance several days, weeks or months, is infradian. For periods of about 1 year's duration circannian rhythm has been used but it is unambiguous to describe these rhythms as annual.

Two basic types of biological time scales can be found in living systems; those that are variable and those that are constant. These may be termed 'physiological' and 'astronomical' time scales respectively. Physiological scales, also described as personal time scales, apply to those rhythms which are a function of the organism or community and do not follow any extrinsic cycle of events. Astronomical or cosmic time scales are governed by the relative positions of the Sun, Moon and Earth, and are applicable to rhythms which are affected directly or indirectly by the external environment (see Part III).

Physiological time scales are variable in that they are specific to one individual and vary between members of a species. For example heart rate depends on a number of morphological and physiological characteristics such as weight to volume ratio, and circulatory efficiency. This does not exclude the rhythm from following cosmic time scales; for example, heart rate follows a circadian and seasonal time scale. Rhythms may, however, depend on external conditions as in the case of the contractile vacuole of protozoa; the periodicity of which depends not only on the rate of discharge and maximal diameter of the vacuole, but also on the osmotic pressure of the surrounding liquid.

Periodicity is often found in the fluctuating numbers of animal communities in competition, notably in the predator/prey relationship. Here special care must be taken in analysis to ensure that cosmic factors play no part. Again the length of this 'ecological' time scale is variable depending upon the resources of the environment available to the community and also on the efficiency of the predator in more complex situations.

The following discussion will deal with those activities of animals which wax and wane repeatedly in a set pattern, occurring one or more times during the life span of the organism. The activities will be considered first at the level of animal behaviour, second in terms of some of their physiological components and lastly, from the viewpoint of the underlying molecular mechanisms. Long-term rhythmical changes in the balance of species, which may be controlled by corresponding climatic cycles, will not be discussed.

Rhythms in behaviour

Animal rhythms may be viewed in two ways. They may be regarded as a series of internal adjustments to cyclic alterations in the physical world. This category of rhythms includes all forms of behaviour which tend to compensate for, or counteract, daily or seasonal variations in light, temperature, rainfall, food availability and nature of the habitat. On the other hand, a large number of rhythms are connected directly with the fact that, for the majority of animals, feeding and reproduction are, fundamentally, periodic activities. It is not easy to classify rhythms in this way, however, because feeding and reproductive rhythms are also synchronized to daily and seasonal changes in the external environment.

General activity

On a daily basis, animal movement is to a great extent linked with the need to discover a food supply. As such, activity cycles are responsible for feeding patterns. The periodicity of movement was one of the first animal rhythms to be examined in detail, partly because it is relatively easy to observe and record 'running activity' in experimental animals but also because man's activities involve an awareness of an internal clock which controls sleep and wakefulness. Quite often human subjects are able to estimate elapsed time very accurately without the aid of mechanical timekeepers. For example, a highly accurate internal 'clock' may operate unfailingly to wake a person a few minutes before a pre-set alarm. Such a regular activity rhythm is said to be under the control of a 'head clock' which may regulate many aspects of behaviour according to a narrowly defined schedule.

   The pioneer experimental work on rhythms in locomotion was carried out by C. P. Richter in the 1920s. Rats were maintained in a laboratory which was darkened between 6 p.m. and 6 a.m. and activity was measured automatically by recording the revolutions of exercise drums attached to the cages. He observed that laboratory rats were active mainly during the hours of darkness although there were considerable variations in the frequency and duration of activity periods during this time interval. Each rat in an experimental group, however, often showed a remarkable consistency in its activity pattern from day to day. Richter found that the periodicity of running activities was markedly independent of the input from sense organs. Neither olfactory nor auditory stimuli were responsible for the rhythm. The role of vision was less clear-cut in that blinding the rats produced variable results. Sometimes there was no effect on the time of onset and duration of running in each 24-hour period, even when observations were continued for many weeks. In other animals the time of onset was delayed by a constant amount each day, and in some it was advanced by a fixed period each day. These deviations in time from the 24-hour cycle varied but did not usually exceed 30 minutes. From day to day there was little variability in the total period of activity for any individual rat. Experiments on several hundred rats showed that they all possessed reliable 24-hour, or nearly 24-hour periodicities in running (Fig. 8.2). The rhythms, whether longer or shorter than 24 hours,

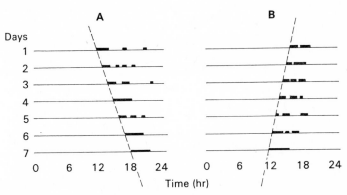

Figure 8.2. Running activity of rodents in continuous darkness. The broken line represents times of onset of activity relative to the experimenter's day. (A) Biological 'clock' starts later each day, indicating that the basic cycle of the 'clock' is greater than 24 hours. (B) Biological 'clock' starts earlier each day, indicating that the basic cycle of the 'clock' is less than 24 hours. In an environment of alternating light/dark each of 12 hours' duration, the 'clock' is synchronized to time of 'lights off'.

did not vary over many weeks by more than a few minutes and were all independent of rhythms in other rats and the immediate environment. All animals showed a close correlation between the frequency of running and the timing of eating and drinking; the usual sequence being running, eating and then drinking. Such a circadian rhythm can be converted into an exact 24-hour rhythm by synchronization with the photoperiod or some other external factor with a 24-hour periodicity.

Little work has been done on the activity patterns of animals in the wild. Recently, however, automatic radiotracking systems have been utilized to record the movements of rabbits and hares. These experiments clearly showed that the onset of activity correlated with sunset and terminated at sunrise and so confirm the laboratory experiments.

Rhythms in humans have been observed with a periodicity of less than 24 hours. For example, subjects confined to bed have activity cycles with a regular periodicity of 1·5–2·0 hours, both when sleeping and awake. In sleeping infants, spontaneous movements have been recorded every 45 minutes. These patterns are probably made up from a complex series of overlapping periodic functions. Sleeping adults, for example, show periods of restlessness which occur at the same time as bouts of contraction of the stomach muscles. In one experiment a subject awoke at the onset of a very large tetanic contraction of the stomach, suggesting that periodic activities of organs may determine overt behaviour.

From training experiments with a number of species it does not appear that periodic activity is based upon the learning of an arbitrary interval of time. Bees, for example, cannot be trained to come regularly for food if the interval between presentation times takes them out of a 24-hour cycle. Further, the activity pattern is determined largely by intrinsic factors and can only be phased by environmental cues. Light is clearly a phasing factor. Laboratory experiments show that the phase setting of activity in day-active animals is partly determined by the change from darkness to light. On the other hand, in a range of nocturnal animals, activity is determined by the time of onset of darkness. Natural conditions never give a sharp cut-off in light intensity. Also, in the wild, darkness and light are not absolute quantities as they are in the laboratory. In keeping with this, it appears that it is the *threshold value* of light intensity which is involved in the precise phase setting of some rhythms. In diurnal crabs, for example, the phasing of locomotory activity is controlled by the relative increase in light intensity at the change from dim to bright light as well as by the *absolute* intensity of the brighter light. Similarly, with some birds in semi-darkness, the brighter the light during the 'dark' period the earlier activity is started.

The light/dark cycle which phases activity rhythms is usually associated with periodic changes in social behaviour. This is most noticeable in certain schooling fishes. For example, the school may disperse at night. This is not simply due to the lack of visual information, but is more concerned with a diurnal fluctuation in readiness to respond to external stimuli. In keeping with this, alerting substances, which evoke cohesion in the school, are more effective in the day-time, even if the fishes are in darkness. This endogenous diurnal fluctuation in 'sensitivity' to the environment may be of widespread occurrence in the animal world. A similar change in social organization is found in littoral crabs which become aggressive in defending territory when exposed to low water but gather together in quiescent groups when submerged.

The natural environment may provide a complex interaction between several variables which makes it difficult to work out the adaptive significance of clear-cut patterns in running activity which are observed in the laboratory. Temperature is one of the environmental factors which clearly influences phasing of activities. This is of particular importance in regulating the behavioural rhythms of reptiles. The ground skink (*Lygosoma*), for example, is active only during the early morning and late afternoon, corresponding to the times when the ambient temperature is between 25 and 30°C. In ants, running occurs later in the day as the temperature increases, and over a moderate rise in temperature, the activity peak may undergo a 12-hour phase shift. Other insects show peaks that are both light and temperature dependent. The fruit fly (*Drosophila*), for instance, exhibits activity phased by temperature at low temperatures and by light at high temperatures.

Environmental factors whose influence are difficult to evaluate concern age, composition of population and the nature of the environment. In the newly emerged dragonfly (*Anax*), a peak of activity occurs at dawn. This peak shifts to midday when the animal is more than a week old. On the other hand, male populations of the fruit fly show two main bouts of activity, both during daylight hours. When males and females are mixed together only one peak occurs, in the dark. With regard to the environment the same species may exhibit different patterns of activity according to its surroundings. For instance the beetle *Feronia* is nocturnal when living in woods but when found in open ground is active mainly in the day. Similarly the biting cycles in mosquitoes vary with habitat. Some organisms exhibit different kinds of activity at different times of the day. Thus, the water-skater (*Gerris*) is found to walk over the surfaces of water in ponds during the daytime but becomes predominantly an aerial form at night. Other insects which fly at night may be swimmers by day. From these observations it is obvious that generalizations are impossible to make with regard to typical rhythms of activity in the wild. It does seem, however, that there is a natural tendency towards multiple rhythms within the 24-hour period, which are not present, or difficult to discern, in the laboratory situation.

Abnormal rhythms in humans

Many psychiatric disorders have been shown to be characterized by long- or short-term rhythms in the appearance of certain clinical features. One of the most exhaustive examinations of institutionalized epileptics has shown that there is a high proportion of epileptics who have a daily fit which occurs at different, but regular times, in each patient. In some patients with various forms of mental illnesses there is also firm evidence for alternating 48-hour cycles; abnormalities appear regularly on alternate days. The symptoms persist for a period very close to 24 hours, with a very rapid transition between the normal and abnormal states. Rhythmical changes in behaviour have also been well documented in schizophrenic patients and in many cases the rhythms were associated with changes in various physiological and biochemical functions.

There is little evidence as to the cause of these abnormal behaviour patterns, which vary from alternating moods of elation and depression to the adoption of specific activities at regular intervals designed to overcome a periodic disability. A number of rhythms appear to be precipitated by illness or accidents that have resulted in a deficiency in an endocrine secretion, and appropriate therapy designed to counteract the deficiency has sometimes resulted in the disappearance of the abnormal behaviour pattern.

Feeding rhythms

The fact that animals have predictable patterns of feeding must have been one of the first facts of natural history observed by man seeking to improve his art of hunting. Two of the most obvious signals for activity in humans are the feelings of hunger and thirst. In this respect, other periodic 'needs' may be established, not connected in an obvious way with the biological purposes of feeding, which involve artificial stimulants; notably cigarettes, alcohol and drugs. Human feeding patterns are obviously conditioned by social demands to a large extent but this training phenomena may be a general feature of animals. Bees, for example, after being offered food for a fixed time for several days will continue to search for food at this particular time even when it is no longer available.

Although feeding activity is to a great extent conditioned by the periodic presence of food, gross periodicities of running in rodents are not markedly affected by food availability. A more fundamental control of feeding appears to be exerted by the nature of the processes of digestion and assimilation. It is probably true to say that feeding is a periodic 'activity' of relative high frequency in most animals. The periodicity may be connected with short-term fluctuations in food supply, perhaps due to rhythmical activity patterns on the part of prey, but is mainly related to the time-lag between food capture and assimilation, which is largely controlled by the speed of digestion. In animals which have the capability of consuming a single large meal in a short time, the common rhythm appears to be feeding leading to satiation with assimilation of the gut contents initiating a new bout of activity. This rhythmical feeding pattern may be evenly spaced over a relatively large proportion of the day. Because 'digestion-time' is related to the amount of food consumed at any one time, the frequency of feeding may vary although the total quantity of food taken per day is maintained at a constant level. Natural frequencies of feeding vary widely from the high level in small birds and rodents, with a high metabolic rate relative to size, to that in some reptiles and fishes which may have a feeding periodicity of days or weeks.

The food gathering activities of most animals appear to be entrained to their photoperiod and are in the main either nocturnal or diurnal. This may be related partly to the relative importance of visual stimuli in detecting food but there may also be a need to use the Sun's position as a direction-finder in animals which undertake relatively long food-gathering migrations each day. Feeding activity may also be synchronized with moonlight. In the nocturnal bee (*Sphecodogasta*), foraging is based on a lunar cycle of 29 days. In the 'crepuscular period' foraging takes place between sunset and the end of twilight. When the Moon is bright foraging activity still occurs providing the 'moonlight' is an extension of twilight.

Although photoperiodicity appears to be the dominant factor in controlling feeding in terrestrial, freshwater and marine organisms, the feeding behaviour of intertidal fauna is also determined by the tidal cycle. The over-riding importance of the tidal rhythms is emphasized by the persistence for some time in the laboratory of rhythms which retain a tidal periodicity. However the blenny (*Blennius* sp.) which is often separated from its food source at low tide, shows no photoperiodic component in movement when examined in the laboratory.

For most littoral animals it is unlikely that activity is bound up absolutely with the state of the tide. Limpets, for example, generally move away from their 'home' depression in the rock soon after being immersed by the incoming tide. The majority of them appear to return to this 'home' after feeding. On the other hand, the animals are also active when exposed, activity being controlled by the period of exposure to direct sunlight and the relative dampness of the environment. However, it seems that tidal rhythms override photoperiod in several shore-dwelling animals. This illustrates the point made previously that for many animals the day-to-day behaviour pattern is controlled by the conditions prevailing in the external environment. This control may be absolute in those animals which are subject to desiccation. Slugs, for example, tend to feed when the humidity rises above a certain level and a species of winkle (*Littorina neritoides*) which occurs up to 7 ft above high water, begins feeding only after heavy rain.

Reproduction

Female rats show a rhythmical rise and fall in running activity superimposed on the normal nocturnal activity cycle (Fig. 8.3). This reaches a peak every 4 or 5 days, corresponding to the physiological events of the oestrous cycle. In many mammals the female is more active than the male, but the obvious behavioural component of the oestrous cycle is the phenomenon of 'heat'. This is the term used to describe the period when the female mammal permits copulation. The oestrous cycle is defined as the time that elapses between one heat and the beginning of the next. Heat denotes the special, usually short-lived, psychological state when the behaviour of the female mammal is distinctly different from that during the rest of the cycle. Indeed the male often shows no interest in females who are out of heat but if a male attempts copulation his advances are repelled.

The underlying physiological cause of the oestrous cycle is the periodic release of hormones from the pituitary gland. However, the physiological events which prepare for possible fertilization of ova are not always accompanied by a clear-cut behavioural rhythm. For example, domesticated animals such as mares and cows occasionally lack the behavioural component of true heat; ovulation occurs but the female is unreceptive to males. This is so-called 'quiet heat'. Sometimes the phenomenon of 'split' heat is observed when the period of sexual receptivity is interrupted by a short period of non-receptivity after which heat is

resumed. A common aberration of sexual behaviour in cattle results in the abolition of the rhythm in mating behaviour. The condition is termed 'nymphomania'
and is characterized by sterility and a continuous manifestation of the psychological desire to mate.

The duration of heat and the intervals between heat vary considerably, even
within the same species, and increasing age generally lengthens the oestrous
cycle. Heat ranges from a few hours (some rodents) to several days, for example,

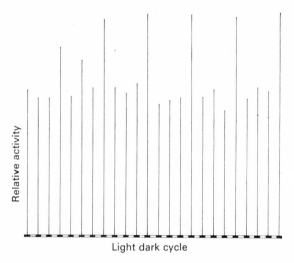

Figure 8.3. Running activity in female rats. Animals shown are active only during
darkness. Dark activity is increased every fourth day, coinciding with the state of
oestrus.

domesticated animals. Sometimes the onset of heat is precisely and regularly
related to the day/night cycle. For instance, some strains of laboratory rats often
mate during the early hours of the morning. There does not appear, however,
to be a periodicity in the desire to copulate in male mammals.

It is only in the primates that periodic sexual receptivity of females is not the
rule. However, there are often subtle changes in behaviour in female primates
which coincide with the menstrual cycle. In humans, depression and mild psychological discomfort sometimes signal the termination of a cycle. Also it has been
noted that the frequency of marital coitus has a marked regularity that is not
equalled in other forms of human sexual behaviour. A maximum frequency is
reached usually during the first two years of marriage then there is a steady
decline. On average the frequency of coitus has been estimated to range from
three times per week for those married in their late teens, to twice per week at
the age of 30 and once per week at 50.

Breeding in man and most domesticated animals takes place throughout the
year. The term 'continuous breeders' has been used to describe these animals.

Some species in this class although they do not have a restricted breeding period show special peaks in fecundity. Man, for example, has distinct annual peaks of prolificacy; in northern latitudes conceptions tend to occur more often in May and June, whereas in the southern hemisphere the corresponding peak is six months out of phase. Similar rhythms in fecundity have been observed in other 'continuous breeders' such as chickens, cattle and rabbits, indicating that 'continuous breeders' have underlying regular or irregular psychological or physiological reproductive rhythms. Seasonal breeders in contrast go through a

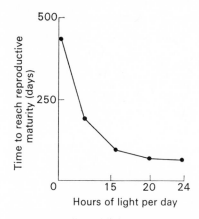

Figure 8.4. Effect of light on sexual maturation in a migratory bird.

definite non-breeding period (anoestrus) during which there are few or no oestrous cycles. It is likely that domestication, with the corresponding tendency for reproductive success to become independent of the food supplies and temperature, was conducive to continuous breeding. It is more usual for animals in the wild to show one or two seasons in the year when reproductive activities occur. During the remaining time, the anoestrous period, the gonads in both males and females may regress and come to resemble those of immature members of the species. Rhythms in behaviour are correspondingly dramatic. Migration is intimately connected with the functional state of the gonads—as is the ritual mating behaviour of many vertebrates.

Reproductive periodicity is controlled undoubtedly in the main by seasonal variations in the intensity and duration of daylight (Fig. 8.4). Despite this, there are basic endogenous rhythms in reproduction seen in 'continuous breeders' under constant lighting conditions which are independent of light. In seasonal breeders an endogenous rhythm may be amplified by a particular change in photoperiodicity to elicit the full reproductive response. Animals may be long-day breeders, where additional light during the non-breeding season accelerates the onset of reproduction, or short-day breeders, which respond to increasing light by decreased reproductive capacity leading to anoestrus. The natural culmination of these rhythms in mammals is pregnancy, during which there is a suspension of the oestrous cycle, although ovulation with a corresponding rise and fall in sexual receptivity may occur. Pregnancy consists of two basic physiological rhythms concerned respectively with gestation (leading to parturition) and lactation.

Breeding behaviour in invertebrates is also controlled through day length. The frequency of mating in invertebrates varies greatly according to species, and it is common to find rhythms in egg laying which are unrelated to mating behaviour. Thus, the desert locust (*Schistocerca*) may mate once and the stored sperm used by the female to fertilize several batches of eggs laid at intervals of about 4 to 5 days. In the milkweed bug (*Oncopeltus*) reproductive cycles take about a day to complete. Mating and feeding occur in the early evening, possibly to allow a maximum opportunity for oviposition and flight during the day. Invertebrates also show migratory sexual behaviour.

Reproductive rhythms in many marine animals are subject to phases of the tides and moon. A most astonishing lunar rhythm is exhibited by the Palolo worm, which inhabits coral reefs in the Pacific Ocean. At the last quarter of the moon in October and November the hinder part of the worm, which is crowded with reproductive cells, breaks off from the foremost part and floats to the surface. Eggs and sperms are shed at low tide on two successive days then this half of the worm dies. Another marine worm (*Odontosyllis*) of the Bermudas, reproduces three times a year; at the first low tide in July, the moon being in its last quarter; then again 26 days later; and after an interval of 26 or 27 days, i.e. late in August. The animals appear on the surface at dusk, usually at about 8 p.m. and become luminescent. At first the female shows no light but suddenly begins emitting whilst swimming rapidly in tight circles. If a male does not appear, illumination ceases after 10–20 sec though the behaviour pattern may be repeated four to five times. The male is also luminous and comes towards the female obliquely from below and heads for the centre of the circle of light. Both animals then swim in a circle together shedding eggs and sperm into the water. This whole behaviour sequence is over by about 8.30 p.m.

Rhythmical behaviour patterns, used to attract male to female, are a feature of many animals. Thus, both sexes of the North American firefly (*Photinus*) emit regular flashes of light. If there is an answering flash within 30 sec after a male emits his flash he will move in the direction of the lure. With large groups of male flies it is often observed that the light emission of all individuals becomes synchronized, giving rise to large pulsating masses of light. Similarly, periodic sounds generated by insects, fishes, birds and amphibians are used as part of the behaviour pattern that leads to mating. Sound production is closely correlated with reproductive behaviour. The male cod produces sounds in the breeding season which stimulate females to participate in breeding. Females are non-vocal at this time. In other species there may be a change in the quality of sound at the onset of breeding. Bird song consisting of a train of phrases repeated at intervals, may be regarded as rhythmical activity. There is a tendency, for instance, to deliver 'syllables' within songs in a rhythmical sequence. Deviations from this order are associated with intervals between syllables which are longer than average. In some birds, singing is common at most phases of the breeding cycle although the nature of the song may vary according to the reproductive state.

Miscellaneous rhythms

Many free-swimming planktonic animals, especially crustacean larvae, undergo characteristic diurnal vertical migrations. Light intensity and wavelength appear to be most important factors in the control of such rhythms, but temperature, gravity, salinity and hydrostatic pressure (discussed earlier, p. 97) may also play a role. Dense accumulations of phytoplankton, however, may tend to disrupt the vertical migration of zooplankton. It is suggested too that many fish, such as, for example, the herring (*Clupea*) may follow their planktonic food source in their vertical movements. The role of photoperiod in entraining vertical migration of the plankton is amply demonstrated in polar seas where vertical migration ceases during the long periods of constant dark and light, but reappears in the spring and autumn.

Many animals undertake periodic long-distance migrations which are entrained to the annual fluctuations in climate. These migrations are governed in the main by extra energy demands perhaps coupled with reproduction. They occur to offset predicted climatic changes and alterations in the abundance of food.

Temperate animals usually become inactive during the winter months when there is a general involution of a number of tissues, particularly the endocrine glands. This is an adaptation to ensure survival during a period characterized by low temperatures and the shortage of food. The reaction entails behaviour patterns which result in the organisms protecting themselves as far as possible from extreme variations in the environment.

An important feature of migration is the ability to measure the passage of time accurately and to couple this with an awareness of a fixed compass point. It is found in crustaceans, insects and members of most vertebrate groups reaching a high degree of development in the migratory and homing birds. This ability to orientate with a 'sun-compass' has been explored with homing insects and birds. In bees it depends primarily on a circadian clock which enables the animal to maintain a constant adjustment to the apparent movement of the Sun (Fig. 8.5).

The periodic renewal of the exoskeleton (moulting) in arthropods is a consequence of the growth process in this group (see p. 122). The actual shedding of the old cuticle (ecdysis) is also linked with changes in behaviour of the organism. Feeding usually ceases sometime before the ecdysis takes place and fixed patterns of behaviour appear. Normal activities are not resumed until the new exoskeleton is firm.

When the mechanism for respiration involves a pumping device for moving the external medium over a specialized body surface for gas exchange, there is clearly a rhythmical muscular movement associated with 'breathing'. As mentioned in an earlier section this activity is continuous in most terrestrial animals

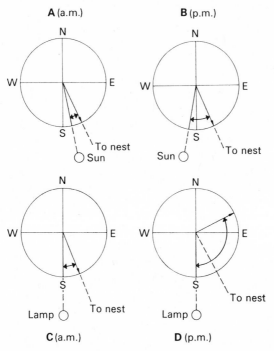

Figure 8.5. Orientation by sun compass. An animal is searching for the SE for nest or food.

A and B The angle between animal and Sun is measured with a built-in correction for the Sun's apparent movement, i.e. the angle allowed increases with the time of day.

C and D If the experimental animal is allowed to orientate with respect to a fixed lamp it still corrects for the Sun but increasingly chooses wrong direction in the artificial environment.

but in some specialized aquatic organisms that inhabit regions low in dissolved oxygen, there is usually a periodic migration of the organism to the atmosphere to take in fresh air and expel the carbon dioxide which has accumulated. These movements are regular, with a periodicity of several minutes and may be observed in certain aquatic molluscs, insects, air-breathing fishes and marine mammals.

Physiological aspects

FEEDING AND GROWTH

All of the rhythmical patterns of behaviour discussed above are characterized by underlying physiological processes which are also of a periodic nature. Those physiological rhythms that have been studied in most detail relate to daily variations in food and water balance and correspond to the feeding pattern.

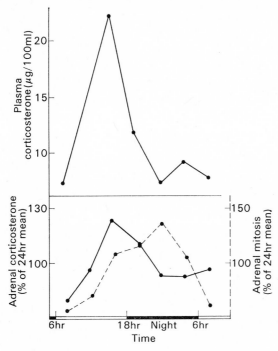

Figure 8.6. Plasma corticosterone in relation to adrenal corticosterone and mitosis in mouse on a 12-hour photoperiod.

They are often heightened in the female during reproduction. In the following discussion most of the illustrations will be drawn from work on the laboratory rat.

Rats maintained under conditions of 12 hours of darkness alternating with 12 hours of light, show a marked diurnal variation in eating and drinking. About 80 to 90% of food and water are consumed during the dark period. There is also a daily fluctuation in the total body weight. In growing animals, a rise of about 7% during the night is followed by a drop of about 4% during the day. The overall weight gain of about 3% per day represents somatic growth. Alongside the periodicities in food and water intake there are corresponding rhythms in evaporative water loss and excretion. Most of the urine, faeces and respiratory water are lost during the hours of darkness. All of these exchanges with the environment imply underlying daily changes in appetite, activity of digestive glands, digestion, assimilation, synthesis of metabolites and kidney function. Many rhythms, in fact, have been observed in laboratory rodents which relate to periodic changes in blood hormones, metabolites and various tissue characteristics (Fig. 8.6). In the kidney, as in other organs, there are diurnal alterations in blood flow. The blood flow and blood space appear to be greatest during the night. This makes it likely that there are corresponding variations in glomerular filtration rate and reabsorption of many components of the filtrate. In this respect, the rhythm in electrolyte excretion in young rats appears to be concerned with the need to accumulate cellular material and expand the extracellular space during the night and reduce the extracellular space during the day.

Daily changes at the physiological level are more difficult to observe in the wild but it has been noted, for example, that there is a periodic alteration in enzyme activity in the digestive tract of intertidal molluscs, which is entrained to the tidal cycle. Intertidal crustaceans have rhythms in total body oxygen consumption which seem to have a tidal basis. Also, wild birds have been found to exhibit diurnal changes in tissue glycogen in keeping with the availability of glucose through the process of assimilation. In this connection one species of weaver, which makes daily feeding migrations over considerable distances from its nesting site, shows a daily rhythm in the mass of pectoral muscle which is utilized as major energy source during the flight.

Many species of mammals show daily cycles in body temperature. The fluctuations may be so great that at the lower temperature the animal may become torpid (Fig. 8.7). Some of these species, in fact, allow the body temperature to fall below those typical of hibernators, yet they cannot survive for long periods at low temperatures. In general, the greatest daily variation in body temperature appears to occur in the smallest mammals. This may be related to the danger these animals encounter as a result of excessive heat loss. Many small mammals become inactive during the winter months and protect themselves through various forms of behaviour against undue heat loss. Non-migratory birds, on the other hand, appear to depend largely upon physiological mechanisms to offset cold weather. They increase their food consumption and, in general through metabolic adaptations, become more resistant to cold. Large seasonal changes in thermal conductivity do not take place. This is in contrast to the rhythms in the growth of fur which are a characteristic of some, but not all, arctic mammals many of which also respond to cold by an elevated rate of metabolism. There are many concomitant adaptations to seasonal changes in temperature at a physiological level. Some of these may not be connected in an obvious way with the need to combat changes in the ambient temperature. In this respect, it has been postulated that the annual rhythm in growth and shedding of antlers in some species of deer is connected with the role of antlers as a heat exchanger.

In poikilothermic organisms many daily physiological rhythms are governed by the changing external environment. The main factor here is the rise and fall in temperature, in as far as it affects metabolic rate. One can appreciate this most with regard to intertidal animals exposed at low water. Water is lost from exposed limpets, particularly those high up on the beach. Even on hot days this loss is well below the lethal level but may reach a value amounting to about 20% of the body weight for animals at the high water mark. When this happens it

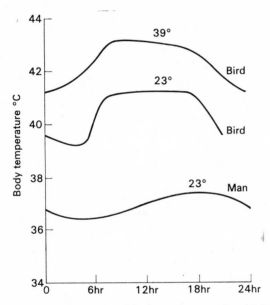

Figure 8.7. Daily cycle of body temperatures in a bird in relation to environmental temperatures compared with that of man.

takes between 3 and 4 hours of immersion for the limpets to recover the lost water. One would expect corresponding daily fluctuations in body fluids and electrolyte balance.

Rhythm is often very well marked in the process of cell-division. In developing eggs of some animals the blastomeres divide at almost exactly the same instant for the first six to seven divisions, resulting in the formation of a perfectly symmetrical hollow ball of cells. From the synchronous nature of mitosis in some mature tissues, one would anticipate that growth would have an underlying 24-hour periodicity.

Periodic changes in growth are most clearly seen as differences in the structure of non-living parts of organisms. For example, examination of the distance apart of external ridges on the shells of clams shows that about five different kinds of striation are formed as the shell is laid down during growth. They have been classified according to their spatial separation. Those furthest apart are interpreted as being due to annual variations and those closer together are thought to represent changes in growth due to equinoctial storms, maximal and minimal amplitude of the tide and diurnal activity patterns.

Growth periodicities longer than 24 hours are not uncommon. For example, structures such as teeth are known to grow in pulses at intervals of several days. A weekly cycle of bone growth has also been described.

The periodic growth of the integument associated with the moulting cycle in the marine decapod crustacea is characterized by marked physiological changes. There is a slow accumulation of reserve metabolites during the intermoult phase; the formation of new cuticle accompanied by resorption of organic matter and salts from the old cuticle during the pre-moult phase; the shedding of the old cuticle, which is associated with a large intake of sea water (amounting to about 65% of the pre-moult weight); and finally, the tanning of the new cuticle and deposition of Ca^{++} salts. There are corresponding changes in the ionic composition of the body fluids. For example, in one species of crustacean the level of calcium at or before ecdysis is said to increase 40–50 times above that at the pre-moult stage.

Periodic loss of part of the integument occurs in the vertebrates, for example, sloughing of the skin in amphibia and reptiles. A process of moulting is found in birds and mammals where there are rhythms in the loss of feathers and hair. (In birds there may be highly localized changes in feather pattern coinciding with the development of semi-bald patches of skin called the brood patches to ensure heat transfer from mother to eggs.) The hair moult cycle has been the subject of much investigation. In rodents there are waves of hair growth which pass over the body surface, there being corresponding rhythms in the activity of the hair follicles. These phenomena are partly under the control of the endocrine system. Long-term hair growth cycles have also been described in fur-bearing animals such as cats and rabbits and in ungulates (see also p. 41).

In sheep it appears that there is an intrinsic rhythm in wool growth which is accentuated by the photoperiod. Fluctuations in wool growth are due partly to seasonal variations in available food and partly to residual variations independent of diet. The latter rhythm is controlled through day-length changes. Normally wool growth is low in winter and high in summer. A reversal of lighting reverses the pattern of growth although this takes about two years to establish. Temperature reversal has no effect.

In addition to changes in the rate of growth it appears that there are also alterations in the characteristics of the growth process. For instance, there is a marked difference in the structure of insect cuticle laid down during the night compared with that synthesized during the day. Chitin in the 'night cuticle' is organized into several layers whilst that in 'day-cuticle' is non-laminate.

Periodicities in the growth process, particularly as seen through rhythms in mitosis, are a common feature of multicellular animals, but it is not established that growth is synchronous in all tissues in the same individual. Changes in photoperiod have been held responsible in cultures of fungi and therefore diurnal growth seems to have been established early in evolution.

REPRODUCTIVE PHYSIOLOGY

Physiological rhythms of reproduction are bound up to a great extent with the need to accumulate energy reserves and protein to sustain the development of gametes and the fertilized ovum. The corresponding physiological mechanisms among seasonal breeders are controlled primarily by an endogenous rhythm which is renewed automatically after each breeding season.

Seasonal accumulations of lipid and carbohydrates are of particular importance in the many animal species where large quantities of eggs and sperm are produced and the feeding and growing phase is separate from the reproductive phase. One of the most detailed studies on the physiology of seasonal reproduction has been carried out on the Pacific Salmon. This animal matures in the sea and migrates hundreds of miles up-river to spawn. During the non-feeding migration, endocrine changes result in the mobilization of muscle protein and lipid stores for the synthesis of eggs and sperm. This species dies after spawning but it is likely that other fishes which undertake several annual reproductive migrations have similar physiological mechanisms. Migrant birds show the same pattern. As they leave their winter quarters, the gonads begin to develop and the plumage starts to take the form appropriate for spring mating behaviour. It is unusual for feeding to take place during the migration and there must be physiological changes in a number of organs due to the internal rearrangement of tissues.

The seasonal utilization of stored lipid is a feature of migrants but is also found in non-migrants. The male pheasant, for example, characteristically loses fat in the spring. Indeed, there is a view that rhythms in vernal fat deposition evolved as a mechanism to take advantage of early seasonal occupancy of a relatively cold environment and that the energy demands of migration may play a secondary role in this adaptation.

It is, however, known that the premigratory build up of lipid deposits is under the control of hormones, principally prolactin. Of great interest in this respect is the finding by Farner that birds seem to possess the ability to 'weigh themselves' and so establish when sufficient fat is present to permit the long migratory flights. This mechanism must involve a delicate sensing of the increment in body weight, possibly through an afferent input to the hypothalamus originating in the neuro-muscular junctions of the wing muscles; for only birds with the opportunity for flight can exhibit the changed behaviour characteristic of the onset of migration. Captive birds without the opportunity for free flight are unable to monitor lipid deposition in this way.

The oestrous cycle in mammals is linked with the cyclic growth and regression of the uterus. Some seasonal breeders show corresponding rhythms in the development of gonads and accessory reproductive structures. There is a fundamental unity here between diverse forms of life, as exemplified by the annual growth and shedding of the antlers of deer and the seasonal growth and loss of the penis in the periwinkle (*Littorina littorea*). The characteristic cycle of placental mammals reaches a peak of expression in the menstrual cycle of primates. Large changes in the cellular organization of the uterus are involved which also entail periodic fluctuations in the work load of other organs. The physiological consequences of the oestrous cycle are particularly dramatic in some female monkeys where the cycle is characterized by the gradual swelling and coloration of the perianal tissues. This rhythm involves the elaboration of mucopolysaccharides which absorb large quantities of water. As the endocrine stimulus of the cycle wanes there is a breakdown of these secondary sexual tissues with the sudden concomitant need for the excretion of a very large volume of water. The rhythmical changes in water balance are associated with large changes in renal function. Another periodic work load is found during lactation. Immediately after birth there is an increase in food and water consumption which coincides with the demand for milk secretion. The increased appetite is manifest in profound changes in the histology and function of the digestive tract. The digestive processes return to normal after weaning.

It is thought that cyclic alterations in endocrine activity are responsible for many rhythmical activities of animals. This is undoubtedly true for reproductive rhythms. In mammals, ovulation occurs at a well-defined time in the oestrous cycle and in primates the ovum is released in response to a rise in the concentration of luteinizing hormone from the anterior pituitary gland. The disrupted follicle in the ovary from which the egg is released develops into a special structure, the corpus luteum, which secretes the steroid hormone progesterone. These changes in the follicle are also brought about by luteinizing hormone. If the ovum is not fertilized the level of luteinizing hormone falls, the corpus luteum regresses and the lining of the uterus regresses, or in the human is shed during menstruation. Fertilization of the ovum results in endocrine changes which initially counteract the fall in luteinizing hormone. The uterus is maintained, the embryo becomes implanted and a new cycle of endocrine events ends with parturition (Fig. 8.8).

A feature of the endocrine system, which is responsible for cyclic activities, is the system of neurosecretory cells. These cells are of nervous origin and are found in the central nervous system. They have the role of converting information from the various sense organs on the state of the environment to specific changes in circulating hormones which co-ordinate the appropriate rhythmical response. From experiments on the cockroach it is suggested that neurosecretory cells in the pars intracerebralis of the brain act as a rhythmic suppressor of locomotory behaviour resulting in a diurnal inactivity. In vertebrates the main neurosecretory transmitting centre lies in the hypothalmic region of the brain. Endogenous rhythmicity in these neurosecretory cells has been implicated in the manifestation of several endocrine rhythms of reproduction. Another important control system in vertebrates centres on the pineal gland. This organ seems to inhibit the maturation of the gonads through the production of the substance melatonin. Light falling on the eyes inhibits the pineal through the sympathetic nervous system and this effect appears to account for the onset of reproduction with increasing photoperiod in a number of vertebrates.

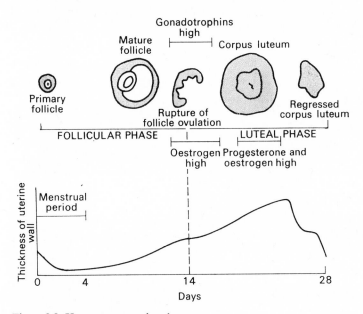

Figure 8.8. Human menstrual cycle.

Physical and chemical models of the molecular clock

Rhythmical phenomena are of great interest to the physicist. Therefore, it is not surprising that many have tried to develop rhythmically functioning models.

A very simple example is the overflow-syphon model which converts a constant process into a rhythmical one (Fig. 8.9). A tap, A, feeds water constantly into tank, C, which can be emptied through a syphon, S, the diameter of which is greater than that of the feed pipe. When the level of liquid reaches the bend in the syphon, it will empty the tank and then shut itself off. The tank will fill up again and if the flow of water from A is constant, the tank will empty rhythmically.

Another classical example is the artificial nerve system proposed by the biologist Lilli. Some iron wires when immersed in concentrated nitric acid, become covered with a coat of iron oxide that protects them from the action of dilute nitric acid. If an electrical or mechanical stimulus is applied to one end of such a wire in nitric acid of specific gravity 1·24, a colour change is propagated along the wire which persists for some time, but finally disappears. This change is due to the formation of the lower oxide of iron which is eventually oxidized. The phenomenon has two things in common with nervous activity. Immediately after the stimulus and lasting until the oxide is converted back to its higher state, there exists a refractory period. Under certain experimental conditions, a permanent stimulus causes a rhythmical activity to appear, chemical changes being propagated along the wire at regular intervals.

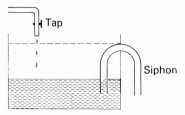

Figure 8.9. Syphon model. The tank is emptied through the syphon when water reaches the level indicated by the dotted line. With a continuous flow through the tap the flow from the tank is periodic.

Electrical models are commonly made in an effort to understand physiological rhythms. One of the simpler circuits consists of a resistance, battery and condenser connected in series, the condenser being shunted by a neon lamp. When the condenser reaches a sufficient terminal voltage, the lamp lights up. This, in turn, short-circuits the condenser which discharges. Then there is a refractory period, during which the battery recharges the condenser until the voltage is again reached.

By connecting up three circuits of this type, it is possible to cause the terminal discharge voltages to build up and discharge in sequence. Also, potential differences could be recorded from this arrangement identical to those obtained from a mammalian heart during activity. Likening the first circuit to the sinus node, the second to auricular tissue and the third to ventricular tissue, it is possible to reproduce the pathological electro-cardiogram changes observed in conduction disorders of the human heart.

Models of this kind are now under intensive investigation within the scientific discipline of cybernetics which deals with the study of control and transmission devices in machines, mechanical and electronic apparatus and human organization. Cybernetics is derived from the Greek word meaning pilot and essentially consists of the analysis of signals and their transmission in electronic and other circuits.

One of the primary ideas of cybernetics of interest in the study of rhythmical phenomena is that described by the term 'feedback' (see p. 6). Certain machines include a sensitive regulating mechanism, arranged in such a way as to ensure steady functioning. When the machine tends to run too fast, the regulating mechanism deducts from the machine a certain amount of energy, reducing its speed. This eventually causes the machine to run too slow and the controller allows extra energy to enter the apparatus. There is an automatic coupling between the work output and energy input to maintain an output which oscillates about the desired mean work output. This kind of feedback system is a feature of most physiological control systems in the body and may underlie some biological rhythms.

However ingenious they may be, these physical models do not explain rhythmical phenomena observed in living organisms. They permit the orientation of research by suggesting working hypotheses or even supplying ideas and provoking thought. This is an undoubted virtue, but it would be a grave error to liken the rhythmical activity of a nerve or nervous circuit to that of a machine or physical model.

Animal rhythms are not merely an expression of multicellular organization. The rhythmical nature of activities at the cellular level impressed the early cytologists. Thus, the contractile vacuoles of protozoa contract at intervals that are often regular. Here, the biochemical events are controlled by rates of ion and water flux across cell membranes. Some protozoa also show a definite cyclic flow of cytoplasm and in certain species the nucleus may be carried rhythmically from end to end of a cell.

Many attempts have been made to elucidate the 'clock mechanism' which underlies animal rhythms at a biochemical level. Although there are clearly regular changes in several enzymes and various cell constituents in step with physiological and behavioural rhythms none of these has been implicated as part of the clock mechanism. The biochemical events seem to be, for the most part, a manifestation of the working of a clock. Thus, in many cases there is no relationship between periodic biochemical changes and the higher rhythms. Also, where such correlations have been established, it has been found that marked, but moderate, interference with biochemical rhythms, using enzyme inhibitors, extra substrate or increased temperature, does not affect the timing at a physiological or behavioural level. On the other hand, drastic interference with metabolism may induce phase shifts. For example, there may be a decrease in the frequency of a rhythm following metabolic poisoning and in some cases the new rhythm may last for several days after treatment.

In the search for a central controlling agency within the cell the nucleus is an obvious candidate. Although there are marked daily changes in the volume of nuclei and the rate of mitosis in animal tissues, there is no direct evidence that this is related to any causal phenomenon. Indeed a few experiments with plants have demonstrated the persistence of rhythms after nuclear metabolism has been inhibited and even after the cell has been enucleated. Against this, some specific rhythms appear to depend upon metabolic processes in the nucleus. This forces the conclusion that there may be a number of different biochemical processes which give rise to clock-like phenomena. The fact that most rhythms at a higher level have been found to be independent of temperature suggests that they are generated either by physico-chemical reactions on membranous structures within the cell, or by diffusion processes associated with ion movement, but at the moment there is no evidence as to the exact molecular mechanism.

Evolution of rhythms

Rhythmical activities are a feature of organisms at every level of organization. Some rhythms appear to be controlled by periodic changes in the external environment. From an evolutionary point of view, the organism must accommodate to these external changes if it is to survive. Therefore the organism responds passively and is adapted to the metabolic consequences. On the other hand, the great proportion of rhythms appear to be inherited and controlled by intrinsic clock-like mechanisms. The simplest interpretation of the adaptive value of intrinsic rhythms is that they alter the behaviour and physiology of the organism in anticipation of a forthcoming change in the environment. In this respect the habitat may be partitioned between many species, which could not co-exist if they were active at the same time, on the basis of their activity rhythms being out of phase with each other. For example, the clock 'tells' an animal what time of day it can expect to meet a mate, catch its prey and avoid falling prey to its enemies. In keeping with this it is often observed that two species have evolved in synchrony; bees, for example, visit flowers only during the hours that they produce nectar. This may involve the development of flexibility of behaviour patterns to ensure learning of a time-sense and the development of orientation devices such as the sun-compass.

Underlying this view we see that the changing external environment also requires the animal to be different in all aspects of its organization as time progresses. Thus, a rat gradually changes from a 'day animal' to a 'night animal' which is totally different in terms of behaviour and physiology. Similarly, where an organism must be able to cope with a wide range of external conditions one could define a species in its summer and winter forms. Also, there may be seasonal demands for the diversion of energy to growth of gametes and young with the 'reproductive form' becoming highly specialized.

During the process of evolution man appears to have become largely independent of intrinsic rhythms as it is advantageous to have the capability of a smooth even performance throughout a 24 hour period. The appearance of pathological rhythms indicates that there is still an inherent rhythmicity which, perhaps by the overlapping of many rhythms, has become obscured. However, man is still dominated by the clock which provides for rest after a period of activity and in this respect he appears to resemble most other multi-cellular animals.

Chapter 9
Seasonal Adaptations

Dormancy

Terrestrial and freshwater habitats differ from the cushioned, relatively constant marine environment in their characteristic instability. During the course of one year, land animals often have to overcome extremes of temperature, humidity and availability of food. The inhabitants of the deeper waters and bottoms of lakes may enjoy a constant temperature, but are nevertheless subject to seasonal fluctuations in the concentrations of oxygen, salts and nutrients. Animals in ponds and small streams may additionally have to suffer periodic desiccation.

It is axiomatic that in the course of evolution all modern animals have become adapted to the exigencies of their physical environment. Polar species grow and reproduce at temperatures which would induce torpor and death in the inhabitants of the tropics. In hot, arid deserts, other species thrive in conditions which would cause lethal heat-stroke or desiccation in animals of temperate regions. Many of these adaptations are discussed elsewhere in this book, but it is worth stressing that the total environment of a particular species includes biotic as well as physical features: the animal's interactions with plants and other animals are as important for its survival as its genetic adaptations to physical conditions. Because of the development of particular morphological, physiological and behavioural features, a species may be well able to withstand the low temperatures of a northern winter, but not the associated shortage of plant or other food.

Development and reproduction proceed normally when environmental conditions are optimal for the species. Unfavourable periods are sometimes surmounted by physiological and morphological changes which may be stressful to the individual and could be damaging to the species. More usually, and particularly when the unfavourable conditions recur periodically, they are avoided by migration or by the intervention of a resting or dormant stage in the animal's life-cycle. Dormancy can involve the suspension of all normal physiological activity in the organism, with a much-reduced metabolism associated with an extremely low level of respiration, and with the development of special adaptations to withstand cold or desiccation. Dormancy may also comprise the suspension of reproductive growth and development, the organism channelling its available resources into the means for staying alive. It can then be difficult to differentiate between the non-breeding periods of species with seasonal reproductive cycles, and the reproductive 'dormancy' of other species. In insects, for example, the suspension of reproductive activity in adults remaining otherwise normal is called gonotrophic dissociation; where the adults also suspend their normal metabolism the condition is considered a true dormancy or diapause. But in mammals, in contrast, seasonal breeding cycles are common, and there is no need to define them as 'gonotrophic dissociation' in comparison with hibernating or aestivating dormancies. Principles and conclusions derived from studies on widely different animal groups often exaggerate the problems of definition. Any such confusion about the definition of dormancy may, perhaps, be resolved in terms of differences in emphasis: the seasonally breeding species have developed adaptations to take best advantage of favourable conditions, whereas species with a reproductive dormancy have adopted mechanisms to avoid unfavourable periods in what would otherwise be a continuous reproductive life.

To avoid successfully a future unfavourable period, its advent must be recognized in advance. It is not surprising, therefore, that migrating species, as well as those with a dormant period, make use of similar predictive environmental clues. Moreover, to take full advantage of the subsequent clement period, the dormant organism must prepare for the ending of conditions unsuitable for development. Here it is likely that animals with a reproductive dormancy will make use of the same environmental tokens as those with seasonal breeding cycles, although species with more deep-seated dormancies may utilize environmental clues for the ending of dormancy which are different from those used for its initiation. The ways in which organisms recognize and interpret the environmental features which signal the approach of inclement and favourable periods during the year are major problems in the understanding of animal dormancy and development.

Many animals react to *immediately* unfavourable conditions by becoming torpid or quiescent. Low temperatures, for example, can reduce the metabolism of a poikilotherm so that its natural physiological processes become impossible. Providing the conditions are not prolonged, recovery rapidly follows their suspension. This quiescence resulting from immediate environmental changes must be clearly distinguished from dormancy, which is induced by environmental changes *in advance* of the conditions which dormancy is designed to overcome. Even so, some homeotherms exhibit daily or periodic torpor which at first sight resembles both the temperature-induced quiescence of poikilotherms and the 'true' torpor of dormancy. Even in some mammals the physiological and behavioural processes which precede dormancy are sometimes omitted in nature, and can be superseded in the laboratory. Only greater understanding of the mechanisms involved in different groups will enable clear differentiation to be made between the various kinds of quiescence, torpor, and dormancy which are known to occur naturally.

In temperate regions, dormancy coincides normally with the inclement winter season and the animals hibernate. But elsewhere, summer may be arid and foodless and the dormant period is an aestivation. Animals in different climatic regions must therefore appreciate signals which indicate the arrival of different seasons, or must react in quite opposite ways to the same signals in different parts of the world. Detailed conclusions about the induction, progress and termination of dormancy are consequently often only applicable to individual species or even smaller inbreeding groups, and generalities may again be difficult to establish.

Dormancy occurs in representatives of almost all living things, from bacteria and protista through most plant and animal phyla, including the angiosperms and the mammals. This suggests immediately that dormancy has arisen many times during evolution, and the formulation of a comprehensive theory of dormancy is made consequently more difficult. However, it is truly remarkable how many animals and plants have adopted mechanisms for the induction and termination of dormancy which are similar in principle although, of course, very different in their fundamental methods of operation.

Dormancy in bacterial and amoebic spores is first indicated by the stimulation of mechanisms leading to the production of structures characteristic of the dormant stage—resistant spore walls, for example—and then by the repression of protein synthesis in the cells. Repression may occur either at the level of transcription (suppression of DNA-dependent RNA synthesis) or translation (enzyme protein production is blocked elsewhere than on the genome—on the ribosomes, for example). Thus the organisms first prepare for dormancy, and then shut down processes involved in energy expenditure.

In the metazoa, particularly the more highly organized forms such as the insects and mammals, preparations for dormancy often include specific patterns of behaviour, the accumulation of food reserves—either within or outside the body—and sometimes the production of structures in which the dormant animal will live. It must be assumed that ultimately the partial inactivation of the genome occurs, and indeed in some species the inhibition of cellular protein synthesis during dormancy is as characteristic as that in bacterial and amoebic spores. But the variety of morphological structure and physiological function in the metazoa imposes an equal diversity in the way in which the final aim of energy conservation is achieved. This account will deal largely with dormancy in insects, a group which offers examples of different kinds of dormancy, but one in which the relationship between the environment and the induction and termination of dormancy can serve as a pattern for the understanding of the phenomenon in other metazoan groups.

Diapause

Insect dormancy is commonly called diapause, a name used originally in insect embryology where it described a stage just prior to the reversal of movement of the embryo round the posterior pole of the egg. The meaning has now altered, and refers to a *condition* of arrested growth, whether embryonic or post-embryonic, rather than to a *stage* of morphogenesis.

Diapause can occur in any stage of the insect life-cycle: in the fertilized egg or in successive stages of embryogenesis; in larval instars; in the prepupal or pupal instars of holometabolous insects; and in the adult instar, especially the female. Normally, diapause intervenes only once in the life-cycle, although exceptions are known, and the particular stage in which diapause occurs is characteristic for the species.

Insect diapause—at least in the pre-adult stages—is a true dormancy, with extremely low metabolic rates and oxygen consumption, complete cessation of development, the assumption of mechanisms to increase cold resistance (including the production of high concentrations of haemolymph glycerol—as effective an anti-freeze in animals as in motor cars!) or resistance to desiccation, the prior production of reserves of proteins and fats, and the development of resistance to infections and chemicals which would be lethal to the non-diapausing insect. Such resistance to infection is found also in hibernating mammals and is probably consequent upon the greatly reduced metabolism of the dormant animal.

Distinction is usually made between 'obligatory' and 'facultative' diapauses in insects. Obligatory diapause is found in univoltine species—those with only one generation each year. Every individual enters diapause, irrespective of the conditions. Facultative diapause, on the contrary, occurs in bi- or polyvoltine species (two or more generations a year), and occurs in nature only in those generations which meet unfavourable conditions. In the laboratory, diapause can be induced or prevented by appropriate manipulation of the rearing conditions. However, with greater understanding of the factors which induce diapause, many examples of apparently obligatory diapause have now been shown to be facultative.

Associated with the physiological preparations for diapause, particular behaviour patterns are shown by many insects. Larvae will seek out hiding places in, for example, the soil, under stones or bark, often reversing their usual reactions to light and gravity. Some species construct special cocoons (hibernacula) in which to diapause. Overwintering pupae of some species have cryptic coloration designed to camouflage them in the absence of foliage. The coloration is specifically associated with the diapausing individuals, and can be quite different from that in pupae of non-diapausing generations. The production of the diapause colour is controlled by hormones, the source of which reacts to the same environmental conditions which will induce diapause. Some adult insects, for example the red locust, remain active during reproductive diapause, but others, such as the Colorado beetle burrow into the soil and become inactive. Yet others, like many ladybird beetles, may migrate to hibernation areas.

THE INDUCTION OF DIAPAUSE

How can insects forecast the approach of unfavourable periods in order to make due preparation for diapause? Since diapause is linked to the cyclic progression of the seasons, it is likely that annual environmental changes are appreciated and interpreted by the pre-diapause insect. Many components of the environment change in a more or less regular manner throughout the year. In summer the average temperatures are high, falling during autumn to their lowest in winter, to rise again in spring. Vegetation goes through a cycle of growth, senescence and decay during the year. Rainfall, air pressure, wind and even light intensity show cyclic seasonal variations. Any or all of these fluctuating environmental factors could be used as clues or tokens signalling the approach of different seasons. But they all suffer from the disadvantages that they are intrinsically variable and changeable from year to year.

One other component of the environment does not have the disadvantage of inbuilt erratic fluctuation: the length of day or photoperiod changes predictably and progressively throughout the year. In high latitudes, daylength varies from 24 hours in the summer to 0 hours in the winter, increasing and decreasing within these limits before and after the summer and winter solstices. At the equator there are 12 hours each of light and darkness throughout the year, and at latitudes intermediate between 0° and 90° N or S, the rate of change of daylength increases with increasing latitude, associated with the longer 'longest days' and shorter 'shortest days' (Fig. 6.4). Thus at a given latitude, there is a regular —and predictable—annual increase and decrease in daylength. Concomitantly, the length of night (the dark period, or scotophase) in every 24 hours varies inversely as the daylength. It is not surprising that many animals have taken advantage of the regularly changing days and nights throughout the year to forecast the onset of seasons favourable or otherwise for growth and development.

PHOTOPERIODISM AND THE INDUCTION OF DIAPAUSE

According to their reaction to daylength, insects with facultative diapause can be classified as long-day or short-day forms. In the former, development is continuous in long photoperiods (or short scotophases) and no diapause intervenes in the life-cycle; exposure to short photoperiods induces diapause in the appropriate stage (Fig. 9.1). The photoperiods over which development will switch from non-diapausing to diapausing may differ by only a few minutes, and it is possible to establish a 'critical daylength' between the slightly longer days which prevent diapause and the slightly shorter ones which induce it (Fig. 9.1.) In short-day insects, long days induce diapause and development is continuous only in short photoperiods (Fig. 9.1). Some insects, particularly those with a true obligatory diapause are photoperiodically neutral while yet others will develop continuously only within severely restricted daylengths—longer *and* shorter days induce diapause. Table 3 gives a list of the photoperiodic reactions of some insects.

Even in latitudes where the annual change in daylength is small photoperiod can still have a regulating effect upon the incidence of diapause. In the red locust (*Nomadacris septemfasciata*) constant photoperiods within 12 and 13 hours in

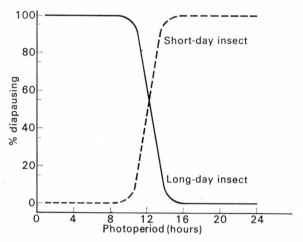

Figure 9.1. Diapause response to photoperiod. Long-day insects are without diapause only at long photoperiods; short-day insects are without only at short photoperiods.

the laboratory (corresponding approximately with seasonal fluctuations in day-length 8°S of the equator) will induce diapause in the adult which lasts 4–5 months. But when the photoperiod is progressively *decreased* from 13 to 12 hours (corresponding to the change in daylength during larval and early adult life in the locust's natural habitat) an adult diapause of 6–8 months is induced. On the contrary, when the photoperiod is *increased* from 12 to 13 hours, dia-pause is eliminated. Thus changing daylength can be as important as the absolute daylength in determining the onset of diapause, particularly where the total fluctuation in photoperiod is marginal.

Of the species so far examined, short-day insects are very much less common than long-day species, and are usually those in which a summer diapause, aestivation, occurs. However, the length of the life-cycle and the developmental stage(s) sensitive to photoperiod are important also in determining whether diapause is a hibernation or an aestivation.

PHOTOPERIODICALLY SENSITIVE STAGES

In order to anticipate the unfavourable conditions which the diapause stage is designed to withstand, the stages sensitive to photoperiod precede usually the diapause stage itself. Thus in the giant silkmoths, *Telea polyphemus* and *Philosamia cynthia*, only the fourth and fifth larval instars react to the short photoperiods which induce diapause in the pupa. In *Antheraea pernyi*, all the larval stages are sensitive to some extent, but the later ones are more so and the effects are cumulative. In *Polychrosis botrana*, the embryo within the egg is most sensitive

Table 3. Diapause stages and photoperiodically sensitive stages in some insect species.

Species	Diapause stage	Sensitive stage(s)	Diapause prevented by
Bombyx mori silk moth	egg	embryo	short days
Pandemis ribeana tortricid lepidopteran	3rd instar larva	1st & 2nd instar larvae	long days
Nasonia vitripennis parasitic hymenopteran	4th instar larva	adult female	long days
Dendrolimus pini pine moth	any larval instar	all larval instars	long days
Pyrausta nubilalis European corn borer	prepupa	late larval instars	long days
Loxostege sticticalis beet webworm	prepupa	late larval instars	long days
Lygaeonematus compressicornis sawfly	prepupa	embryo	long days
Abraxas miranda geometrid lepidopteran	pupa	early larval instars	short days
Pieris brassicae cabbage white butterfly	pupa	4th & 5th larval instars	long days
Polychrosis botrana grape berry moth	pupa	embryo (+1st larval instar)	long days
Telea polyphemus polyphemus moth	pupa	4th & 5th larval instars	long days
Leptinotarsa decemlineata Colorado beetle	adult	late larval instars+adult	long days
Anopheles maculipennis malaria mosquito	adult	late larval instars+adult	long days

to light, the first three larval stages less so, to induce a pupal diapause. In the Colorado beetle (*Leptinotarsa decemlineata*) which has an adult diapause, the larval stages are sensitive to light together with the adult itself, and in *Dendrolimus pini*, with a larval diapause that can occur in any stage, the larvae themselves are sensitive to light. Certain races of the silkmoth (*Bombyx mori*) show the opposite extreme, in which the embryos developing in the egg of one genera-tion are sensitive to photoperiod and temperature to induce diapause in the eggs of the next generation. Most insects react to the blue-violet end of the spectrum as they do to white light; the long wavelengths having the same effect as darkness. This is quite opposite to the situation in most plants. The Colorado beetle and *Acronycta rumicis*, however, react photoperiodically to the whole spectrum.

The number of instars, together with the lapse of time, between the photo-periodically sensitive stages and the diapause stage thus determine whether the diapause is a hibernation or an aestivation. In typical long-day species of north temperate regions, development during the shortening days of late summer induces subsequent hibernation. But in the univoltine jassid, *Stenocranus minutus*, a short-day species, development during the long days of early summer induces a prolonged adult diapause, which includes hibernation. Conversely, in the bivoltine race of the short-day *Bombyx mori*, in which almost a whole generation elapses between the photoperiodically sensitive embryonic stages and the diapausing egg of the following generation, development during the short days of late winter and spring prevents diapause in the subsequent eggs, whereas embryonic development during the long days of summer causes the next genera-tion of eggs to enter a hibernating diapause.

PHOTOPERIODISM AND TIME MEASUREMENT

The stage(s) sensitive to photoperiod in an insect's life-cycle frequently shows a characteristically sharp change in response around the critical daylength (Fig.

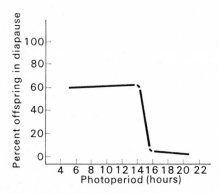

Figure 9.2. The effect of photoperiod on the production of diapause larvae by females of *Nasonia vitripennis*, showing the abrupt change at the critical daylength. (After D. S. Saunders (1969) *Symp. Soc. exp. Biol.* **23**, 301–329.)

9.2), the difference of even a few minutes determining whether or not there will be a subsequent diapause. This suggests that the insect has the capability of measuring accurately the length of the light period, the dark period, or both. To do this, the insect must make reference to some internal or physiological rhythm.

Circadian rhythms have been mentioned elsewhere (p. 133), and clearly could provide a reference for measuring the light and dark periods during the progression of the (almost) 24-hour cycle. It must be remembered, however, that other time-measuring devices exist—the egg-timer or hourglass type is the most obvious. If an endogenous process taking a precise interval of time to complete were triggered by the onset of the photoperiod, or by the scotophase, then the lengths of the light or dark periods could be assessed by comparison with the time of completion of the process.

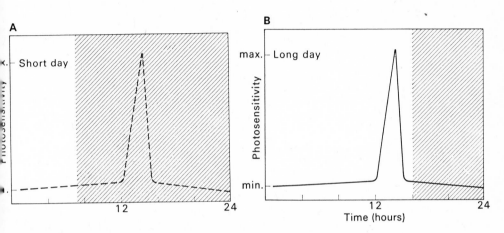

Figure 9.3. Relationship between photosensitivity and day length. (A) The days are too short to overlap the maximum photosensitive period and diapause results. (B) The long day overlaps the peak of photosensitivity, the photoinducible process is stimulated and diapause is prevented.

There is evidence that both circadian rhythms and interval timers are used in different species for measurement of the light/dark cycles. It can be difficult to distinguish between them, because it must be assumed that in nature both mechanisms have become adapted to the normal 24-hour environmental cycle. In the laboratory, 'days' and 'nights' of unnatural lengths can be employed, and 'nights' of normal lengths can be scanned by periodic light flashes. The results of these experiments suggest that some insects 'measure' the length of the dark period, whereas others show a circadian rhythm of 'photoinducibility' with maximum sensitivity occurring a definite time after the previous 'dawn' or 'lights on', and sometimes with a second peak of sensitivity a certain time before 'dusk' or 'lights off'. If the photoperiod or daylength is sufficiently long to coincide with the photoinducible maximum, then diapause is prevented and direct development ensues. If the days are too short to overlap the photoinducible peak, then direct development is prevented and diapause results (Fig. 9.3).

It should be stressed that the phenomenon of circadian photosensitivity in insects is not concerned solely with diapause induction and prevention. Adult emergence rhythms, locomotory rhythms, oviposition rhythms, and so on, can all be governed by such a mechanism. The widespread nature of the phenomenon is accentuated when it is remembered that dormancy and flowering in plants, migration in birds and fish, reproductive rhythmicity in many vertebrates and invertebrates, are all associated with the appreciation and interpretation of photoperiod.

TEMPERATURE AND DIAPAUSE

It was once thought that high temperatures prevented and low temperatures induced diapause through effects upon the metabolism of insects. But it is now accepted that temperature acts as a signal for the induction or otherwise of diapause in much the same way as the photoperiod stimulus. In general, temperature and photoperiod interact in such a manner as to support or nullify the

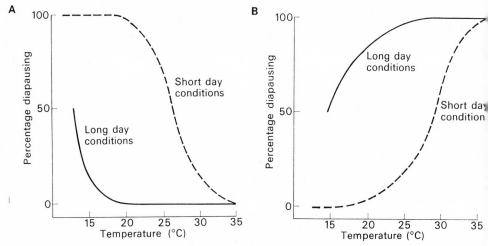

Figure 9.4. Relation between temperature and daylength in inducing diapause. (A) For a long-day insect, low temperatures will induce diapause even in long-day conditions, whereas higher temperatures offset the effects of short-day conditions. (B) For a short-day insect, low temperatures can offset the effect of long-day conditions, whereas high temperatures will induce diapause even under short-day conditions.

tendency to diapause. Thus in long-day insects, high temperatures support the effects of long photoperiods in preventing diapause, and low temperatures strengthen the effects of shorter photoperiods in inducing diapause. In short-day insects, on the contrary, low temperatures act with short photoperiods to prevent diapause and high temperatures with long photoperiods to induce diapause (Fig. 9.4). Under natural conditions, of course, higher temperatures are associated usually with longer days, and presumably insects have become adapted to these combinations.

In the laboratory, extremes of temperature at the 'wrong' times in an insect's life-cycle can have remarkable effects. Thus chilling at temperatures just above freezing for a few hours every day at different times in the light/dark cycle can reverse the normal photoperiodic effects on diapause induction, particularly if the photoperiod is close to the critical daylength (Fig. 9.5). This can be ex-

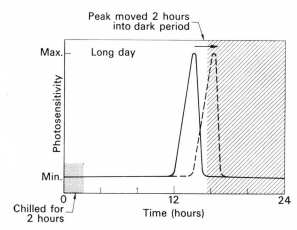

Figure 9.5. Effect of chilling at the beginning of the light period in a long-day insect reared in long days. The photoinducible mechanism is moved an equivalent two hours into the dark period and is thus not stimulated and diapause results.

plained by supposing that chilling slows down or stops the time-measuring process, whether circadian clock or interval timer, so that the photoinducible peak is brought out of phase with that occurring at normal temperatures. Chilling would thus have the overt effect of shortening the light or the dark period, depending upon when it is applied, thus converting the effect of photoperiod from long to short day or *vice versa*.

OTHER FACTORS AFFECTING DIAPAUSE

Poor quality and insufficient quantity of food, lack of water, the age of the mother (particularly in egg diapauses), and the physiology of the host in diapausing parasites may all affect the incidence of diapause in different insect species. One or other of these factors may be of greater importance in diapause induction in some insect species than in others. Overall, they act to modify the effects of the primary tokens of photoperiod and temperature, and are perhaps of greatest significance around the period of critical daylength. In nature, food and water resources vary usually in relation to the season, and the insect's responses to their fluctuations will be adaptive in the same way as to photoperiod and temperature. The whole environment can thus contribute to the determination of diapause, and its exact time of onset can be varied slightly so that advantage can be taken of 'good' years, and 'bad' years will promote and strengthen diapause in the population.

Although photoperiod is the primary token in inducing diapause, its termination is controlled in most insects by temperature. In temperate species, temperatures lower than those necessary for normal metabolism and development are effective in bringing diapause to an end, although the most effective temperature ranges vary with the species. Thus the optimum temperature for diapause termination in the eggs of the silkmoth (*Bombyx mori*) is about 7°C; in diapause eggs of *Austroicetes cruciata* it is about 10°C. Diapausing pupae of *Smerinthus ocellatus* will reinitiate development when kept at temperatures just above freezing; pupal diapause in *Hyalophora cecropia* is most effectively terminated by temperatures of 10–15°C. Insects from warmer climates have optimal temperatures for diapause termination higher than those from temperate regions: diapause in the eggs of the cricket, *Gryllulus commodus*, is terminated at a temperature range extending from 8 to about 27°C, with maximum effectiveness at about 13°C; egg diapause in the brown locust (*Locustana pardalina*) is terminated by temperatures as high as 35°C; adult diapause in the Colorado beetle is extended by low temperatures, but termination is accelerated at a temperature of 30°C.

Diapause is brought eventually to an end when the insects are kept at temperatures on either side of the optimum, but below particular minimum and above maximum limits, diapause will continue. Moreover, a minimum period of time even at the optimum temperature is necessary before diapause is terminated, and this period becomes more extended at temperatures within the range on either side of the optimum (Fig. 9.6). This indicates clearly that diapause is not 'broken' by temperature 'shocks' as was at first thought. The requisite temperatures for the most effective termination of diapause must be necessary for the completion of some temperature dependent process which will bring diapause to an end. The process may be called diapause development, and progresses most efficiently at the optimum temperature while taking longer at temperatures other than the optimum, and proceeding not at all at temperatures outside a particular range.

Once diapause has been brought to an end, the temperature optimum for normal growth and development may be very different from that for diapause development, and in temperate regions is usually higher. But normal development can take place at a range of temperatures on either side of the optimum, and if this range overlaps that for diapause development then diapause termination, followed by normal growth and development, can occur at temperatures intermediate between the optima for the two processes (Fig. 9.7). But if the two temperature ranges do not overlap, then neither diapause development nor post-diapause development will proceed at temperatures intermediate between the two ranges. The temperature requirements for diapause and post-diapause

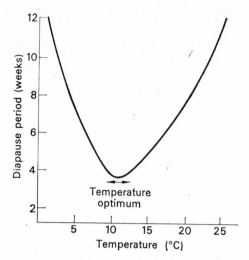

Figure 9.6. Relation between diapause development and temperature. Although diapause can be terminated at a range of temperatures on either side of the optimum, the process takes considerably longer.

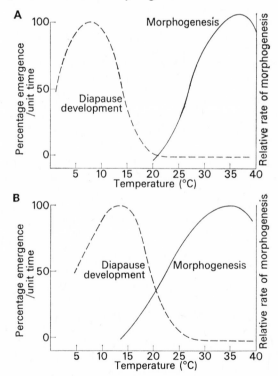

Figure 9.7. Relation between temperature requirements of diapause development and subsequent morphogenesis. (A) The range of temperatures over which diapause can be broken does not overlap with that necessary for morphogenesis: consequently temperatures between the two optima will not allow development. (B) Temperatures within the range 15–25°C will allow slow diapause development *and* morphogenesis.

development can, therefore, be of critical importance in limiting the geographical distribution of an insect species. There is evidence, however, that species with wide geographical distributions are divided into 'physiological' races, with different temperature requirements for diapause development and even with different critical daylengths for the induction of diapause: the possibility of adaptation to different environmental conditions must never be discounted.

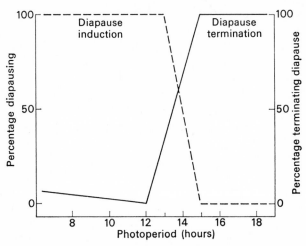

Figure 9.8. Relation between diapause induction and termination in *Antheraea pernyi* pupae. Photoperiods which prevent diapause induction are similar to those which terminate diapause in previously chilled pupae. (After C. M. Williams & P. L. Adkisson (1964). *Biol. Bull. mar. biol. Lab., Woods Hole*, 127, 511.)

Although temperature is of prime importance for diapause development, photoperiod plays also a part in the termination of diapause in some species. Thus the silkmoth, *Antheraea pernyi*, exposed to a temperature of 2–3°C for five months or more will terminate its pupal diapause. But if the pupae are subjected to the low temperature for 8–11 weeks and are then placed at 25°C in photoperiods greater than about 15 hours, diapause is brought rapidly to an end. Photoperiods shorter than about 13 hours have no such accelerating effect upon the termination of diapause; in fact, the photoperiods which act upon the sensitive larval stages to induce diapause in the subsequent pupal stage are the same as those which maintain diapause in the pupa. Similarly, the photoperiods which prevent diapause are the same as those which terminate diapause in the pupa (Fig. 9.8). The critical daylength for the induction of diapause is similar to that for the termination of diapause (Fig. 9.8).

ENDOCRINOLOGY OF DIAPAUSE

In insects, growth, moulting and development are controlled by the synergistic action of two hormones: ecdysone and juvenile hormone (Fig. 9.9). The hormones are secreted by epithelial endocrine glands—ecdysone from the thoracic glands or their equivalents, and juvenile hormone from the corpora allata (Fig. 9.10). The activity of these glands is controlled by trophic hormones secreted by specialized nerve cells in the brain, the neurosecretory cells (Fig. 9.10). The thoracotrophic hormone passes along the neurosecretory axons to be released from axon terminals in the corpora cardiaca; the allatotrophic hormone(s)

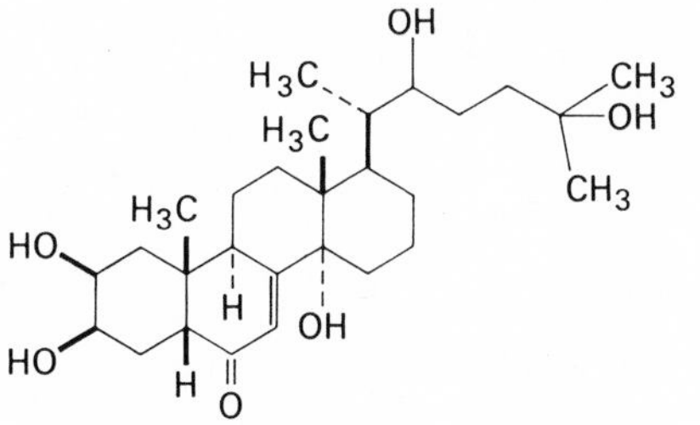

α-ecdysone
(2,3β,14α,22R, 25 − pentahydroxy -Δ7-5β-
cholesten-6-one)

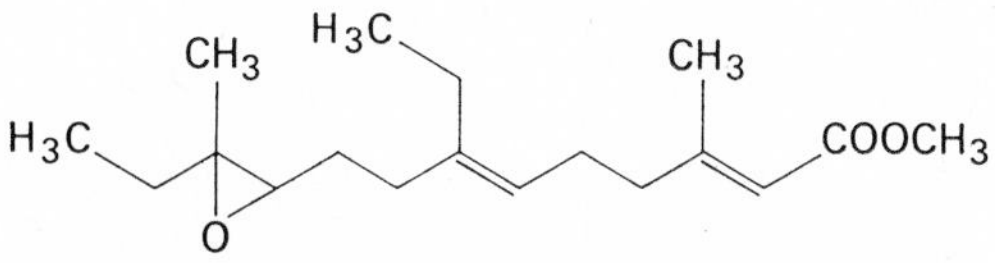

Juvenile hormone
(methyl 10-epoxy-7-ethyl-3, 11-dimethyl-
2,6-tridecadienoate)

Figure 9.9. Ecdysone and juvenile hormones.

travel along the neurosecretory axons directly to the corpora allata (Fig. 9.10). The corpora cardiaca are highly specialized parts of the dorsal sympathetic nervous system, with which they remain in nervous continuity (Fig. 9.10). In addition to acting as sites for the storage and release of cerebral neurosecretory hormones, the corpora cardiaca produce their own intrinsic hormones. In some insects, there is evidence for the presence of both stimulatory and inhibitory allatotrophic hormones, so that the activity of the corpora allata can be very closely controlled. Neurosecretory hormones, together with intrinsic hormones from the corpora cardiaca, also control many of the intermoult activities of cells and tissues.

In adult pterygote insects, the thoracic glands regress and disappear during or shortly after the moult to the adult, and consequently the adult insects do not moult. In many insects the corpora allata are involved in the control of reproduction, particularly vitellogenesis. The cerebral neurosecretory cells with their associated corpora cardiaca play also an important part in this control, both by the continued production of allatotrophic hormones and by the secretion of hormones which are involved in the vitellogenic process.

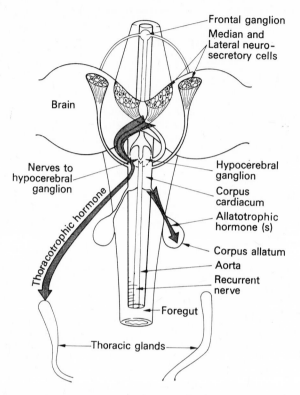

Figure 9.10. Diagram of the insect endocrine system, showing particularly the relationship between the cerebral neurosecretory cells and the corpora allata and thoracic glands.

There is now overwhelming evidence that the immediate cause of diapause is a change in the endocrine status of the insect. Pupal diapause in *Hyalophora cecropia* results from the non-production of thoracotrophic hormone by the cerebral neurosecretory cells with consequent lack of activation of the thoracic glands. Diapause development at low temperatures is associated with the attainment of 'competency' of the brain to produce its hormone, and hormone release occurs during the subsequent period at the higher temperature. The effect of the low temperature in terminating diapause is entirely upon the brain: chilled brains implanted into an unchilled pupa will terminate diapause. Injections of ecdysone will also bring diapause to an end in unchilled pupae whose brains have been removed. Indeed, ecdysone injected into isolated abdomens of diapausing pupae will terminate diapause and initiate complete adult development, including the production of viable eggs.

In *Antheraea pernyi*, the modifying effects of photoperiod upon diapause development initiated by previous low temperatures also operate directly upon the brain. Brains transplanted to the tip of the abdomen underneath a perspex disc will react to photoperiod in the same way as those *in situ* under the transparent cuticle of the head. Brains from which the neurosecretory cells have been removed do not terminate diapause, and it is likely that photoperiods of the appropriate lengths affect the transport and release of thoracotrophic hormone.

Pupal diapause thus results from changes in the normal cycle of production and release of a major developmental hormone—the thoracotrophic hormone from the cerebral neurosecretory cells. It is likely that pre-pupal and larval diapauses are controlled in a similar manner, for the thoracic glands are inactive during diapause in these stages also. However, larval diapause in the rice stem borer (*Chilo suppressalis*) is correlated with the continuous secretion of juvenile hormone by the corpora allata. It is not clear how a high titre of juvenile hormone affects the incidence and maintenance of the larval diapause in this species, for in some other insects, juvenile hormone will activate the thoracic glands and in others stimulates the synthetic activities of the cerebral neurosecretory cells. The endocrine basis for diapause in *Chilo suppressalis* underlines the importance of the target tissues in all endocrine mediated processes: in this instance, juvenile hormone may programme the tissues for diapause in the same way that it programmes them for other developmental routes. It must be assumed that in any diapause, when the cells of the body react to changes in the hormone balance by entering a developmental arrest, this reaction is itself adaptive and must be imprinted in the genome.

Adult diapause is associated also with changes in the balance of developmental hormones in the body, but here the hormones are those normally concerned with the control of reproduction. In the Colorado beetle, juvenile hormone is absent or present in minimal concentrations during diapause. All the symptoms of diapause—behavioural as well as developmental—can be induced in otherwise non-diapausing individuals by removal of the corpora allata. In the bug *Pyrrhocoris apterus*, the reduced oxygen uptake of diapause can only be achieved in non-diapausing individuals if the corpora cardiaca as well as the corpora allata are removed. In this species, therefore, the cerebral neurosecretory system as well as the corpora allata is involved in diapause. In the Egyptian grasshopper (*Anacridium aegyptium*) there is also evidence that inactivity of the cerebral neurosecretory system, together with the corpora allata, is associated with adult diapause. It is possible, therefore, that in adult, as well as larval and pupal diapauses, the prime mover in inducing and maintaining the developmental arrest is failure of the brain to produce or release its hormones.

Diapause in larvae, pupae and adults thus results from the absence of specific developmental hormones. Egg diapause, on the contrary, is induced by the presence of a diapause hormone. In the silkmoth (*Bombyx mori*) the hormone is manufactured by a pair of neurosecretory cells in the sub-oesophageal ganglion, produced and released during the pupal period after adult development has been initiated. The oocytes take up the hormone during a particular stage in their development. In individuals destined to produce diapause eggs, the production and release of the hormone by the suboesophageal neurosecretory cells is stimulated apparently by nervous impulses arising in specific centres in the brain and travelling to the sub-oesophageal ganglion *via* the circum-oesophageal commissures (Fig. 9.11). In individuals producing non-diapause eggs, on the

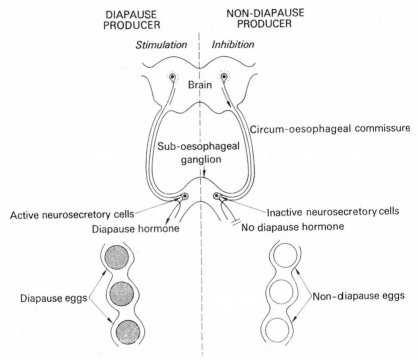

Figure 9.11. Diagram of the nervous and endocrine mechanisms involved in the production of diapausing and non-diapausing eggs of *Bombyx mori*.

contrary, the production and release of the hormone is inhibited by nervous impulses from the brain (Fig. 9.11). Consequently, severing the circum-oesophageal commissures or implanting sub-oesophageal ganglia will promote the production of mixed diapause and non-diapause eggs in both diapause producing and non-diapause producing individuals—in the former because the stimulus for full production of the diapause hormone is absent, and in the latter because the inhibition on diapause hormone production is lifted (Fig. 9.12). The proportion of diapause to non-diapause eggs produced will depend both upon the length of time elapsed after pupation before the operations are performed, and upon the time of maximal uptake of the hormone by the sequentially developing oocytes.

At the cellular level, diapausing pupae of *Hyalophora cecropia* respond to the presence of adequate concentrations of ecdysone by increased *m*-RNA synthesis, accompanied perhaps by the activation of existing 'long-lived' *m*-RNAs. It is uncertain where in the cell the hormone acts to produce these effects. In other insects, favoured hypotheses suggest the nuclear membrane or the genes themselves is the site but the re-establishment of cellular protein synthesis is a *sine*

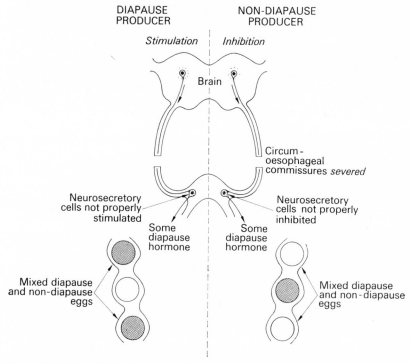

Figure 9.12. The effects of severing the circum-oesophageal commissures (or of removing the brain) upon the production of diapausing or non-diapausing eggs in *Bombyx mori*.

qua non for diapause termination and further development. In adult *Leptinotarsa decemlineata* the haemolymph proteins of diapausing and non-diapausing individuals are different in number and kind, suggesting again that the altered endocrine balance of diapause affects the protein synthetic machinery of cells— presumably the fat-body for haemolymph proteins, but also the flight muscles and ovaries in the Colorado beetle. Diapause eggs of *Bombyx mori* contain more glycogen and lipids than non-diapause eggs, and also larger quantities of 3-hydroxykynurenine associated with the formation of the ommochrome pigment which differentiates the two kinds of egg. The diapause hormone in *Bombyx mori* affects that stage in the development of the oocyte when the nurse cells degenerate and follicle cells surround the oocyte and one result of its action is increased trehalase activity, so that larger quantities of blood trehalose are utilized for glycogen formation in the oocyte. This incidentally has a feedback effect upon other tissues in the pupa, inducing changes in the metabolism of lipid, protein and carbohydrate. The effects of the diapause hormone upon enzyme activities in the follicle cells and oocytes must be mediated by the protein synthetic machinery of the cells, although how the subsequent diapause is induced is unclear. These changes in metabolism associated with diapause egg production can be compared with pre-dormancy metabolism in bacterial and amoebic spores, and with the pre-diapause preparations characteristic of the post-embryonic diapauses in many insects. The virtual cessation of cellular protein synthesis in diapausing pupae, for example, is comparable with that of dormant spores. There can be no doubt that the fundamental mechanisms of dormancy in other organisms are paralleled by at least some diapause processes in insects.

STORAGE OF ENVIRONMENTAL INFORMATION

Although much is known about the endocrine basis of diapause in different stages in insects, many problems remain. Thus although the relationship between photoperiod and diapause is well established, knowledge about the sites of photoperiodic reception is fragmentary. Surprisingly, the compound eyes and ocelli seem not to be involved in photoperiod appreciation. In pupae of *Antheraea pernyi*, neurones close to the medial neurosecretory cells in the brain appear to be receptors for photoperiod, and in other insects neurones elsewhere in the central nervous system seem to be responsible. A major problem is revealed when it is remembered that the stages sensitive to photoperiod are often separated from the diapausing stage by several intervening instars. Since post-embryonic diapause in many insects involve the switching off of cerebral hormone production, which must function normally to control growth and development in the intervening instars, how is the environmental information stored between the sensitive and diapause stages? How is the endocrine system switched off when the appropriate time for diapause arrives? In *Antheraea pernyi* pupae, the whole complex for photoperiod appreciation, time estimation, and the mechanism for inducing the transport and release of neurosecretions, all seem to reside in those parts of the brain in close proximity to the medial neurosecretory cells. Whether similar situations obtain in other insects is unknown. In *Bombyx mori*, photoperiod and temperature affect the developing embryo so that diapause is induced or prevented in the eggs of the subsequent generation. How this environmental information is appreciated and translated into mechanisms for the stimulation or inhibition of diapause hormone production at the appropriate time by the pupal sub-oesophageal ganglion, remains a central problem in the understanding of diapause.

Breeding experiments, for example, between diapausing and non-diapausing races of *Bombyx mori*, have demonstrated quite clearly that diapause has a genetic basis. Several genes are involved in the inheritance of diapause, which are probably associated with variability in the receptor mechanisms for environmental information, in time estimation and 'counting' processes, and perhaps also in the reaction of the endocrine system to its integrated stimuli. The establishment of 'physiological' races in an insect species, in which the diapause response to environmental tokens may vary, is thus no more surprising than the development of the more familiar morphological and chromatic varieties.

Hibernation

As noted earlier, very many vertebrate animals have seasonal breeding cycles. In the non-reproductive times of the year, they exhibit a form of gonotrophic dissociation, which may be considered similar to that found in some adult insects when environmental conditions are less favourable for reproduction or feeding the young. But whereas gonotrophic dissociation in insects is thought of as a form of diapause, seasonal breeding in vertebrates is so commonplace that it excites no comment. The difference in emphasis no doubt lies in the relative lengths of the life-cycles in the two groups: the rapid development of insects during one year or part of the year makes the delayed or interrupted reproduction of a few species unusual and obvious; in vertebrates, on the other hand, with life-cycles frequently extending over several years, reproductive arrest for periods of the year is to be expected.

The periods of reproduction in many vertebrates are controlled by the photoperiod. Long-day and short-day species are known, and the principles of estimating daylength by correlating photoperiod and/or scotophase with an internal clock—either an interval timer or a circadian rhythm (see also p. 137)—are as well established in vertebrate animals as in insects. It is perhaps only in the amphibians that the photoperiod 'sense' is poorly developed.

The environmental control of reproduction affects ultimately the production of gonadotrophic hormones by the anterior pituitary, mediated by the hypothalamo-hypophysial neurosecretory system which produces the specific gonadotrophic releasing factor (Fig. 9.13). The pineal gland, at least in members of some vertebrate classes, plays a part in mediating the effects of environmental light—perhaps as part of the 'counting' system—and in some way affects the production of the hypothalamic hormones.

In some birds and fish, reproduction frequently alternates with migration so that unfavourable seasons are avoided. Some mammals migrate for the same reason, but a few species avoid the unfavourable season by either aestivating or hibernating. In migrating birds, the restlessness which culminates in migration (both away from and back to the breeding areas) is controlled precisely by daylength. In hibernating mammals, on the contrary, temperature plays the predominant part in entraining the hibernating torpor, although the alternation of reproductive activities, controlled by photoperiod, with dormancy suggests that daylength has an effect here too, albeit less importantly. It is most likely that photoperiod assumes greater importance when extensive preparations for dormancy have to be made.

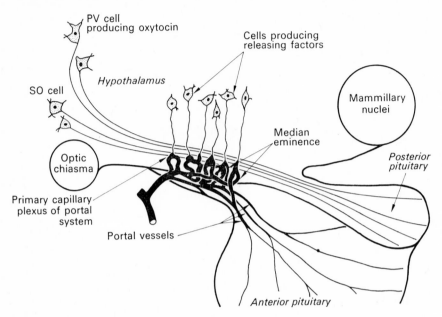

Figure 9.13. Diagram to show relationship of nervous control of the posterior pituitary and neuro-humoral control of the anterior pituitary in the median eminence of the hypothalamus. The axons of the neurosecretory cells of the paraventricular (PV) and supraoptic (SO) nuclei pass without interruption to the posterior lobe of the pituitary where their hormones are discharged into the general circulation. The anterior pituitary is controlled by releasing factors produced by neurones in the hypophysiotrophic area of the hypothalamus and discharged into the primary capillary plexus of the portal system. (From B. A. Cross in *Hormones in Reproduction.* Ed. C. R. Austin & R. V. Short. Cambridge University Press.)

Most mammals known to be deep hibernators belong to the orders Insectivora, Chiroptera and Rodentia, of which the rodents include by far the largest number and variety of hibernating species.

Mammalian hibernation differs from insect diapause in that the profound torpor of hibernation can be interrupted by short periodic arousals throughout the colder months, arousals which increase in frequency towards the end of the hibernation period. Moreover, some mammals make 'test drops' into torpor at the approach of the hibernation season, brought on by reducing temperatures but from which the animals recover quickly before entering their true hibernation. Some bats have a diurnal rhythm of torpor, and the ways in which the various kinds of torpor are related are obscure. Nerves and certain muscles retain their functions at the markedly reduced body temperatures of hibernation, although this is also characteristic of animals living in arctic regions.

The relationship between hibernation and reproduction is well illustrated by the hedgehog and many rodents. In the females, a period of anoestrus begins in the autumn and extends throughout the hibernation period which begins a little later. The end of hibernation in spring is followed closely by reproductive activity, and insemination through to rearing the young takes place before the next hibernation. In many bats, on the other hand, oestrus and copulation occur in the autumn, and all subsequent phases of the cycle (ovulation, fertilization, pregnancy and lactation) are held suspended during hibernation and are resumed in the spring. The long-lived viability of the sperm within the reproductive tract of the female is not necessarily due merely to the low temperatures of hibernation, although how the sperm are enabled to live for these periods of time is unknown. In the bats, *Miniopteris schreibersii* and *M. australis*, copulation, fertilization and the first stages of embryogenesis take place before hibernation. There is no development beyond the free blastocyst stage in the uterus, and implantation and true pregnancy do not occur until after arousal from hibernation. Such delayed implantation is well known in other non-hibernating mammals, where it is a clear response to photoperiod and is a means of prolonging pregnancy over the less favourable months of the year. Whether such delayed implantation in these two species of bat is also a photoperiodic response, or whether a different environmental token such as temperature provokes the response is not known.

Preparations for hibernation include the functional involution of the anterior pituitary and other endocrine glands directly dependent upon it, with the exception perhaps of the adrenal cortex and, in female bats, the gonads. Other endocrine glands not controlled directly by the adenohypophysis, such as the adrenal medulla, may show an accumulation of secretion which is discharged during temporary arousals. Accumulations of neurosecretion in the hypothalamus and posterior pituitary have been described in some hibernators, and it must be supposed that the release of hormones controlling the adenohypophysis is suppressed.

Many small mammals have the ability to rewarm themselves spontaneously, even when their body temperatures are cooled to as much as 20°C below normal. This ability is developed best in hibernating species, which can rewarm themselves from lower temperatures even in the summer when they are not in hibernation. Spontaneous rewarming may be associated with the presence of brown fat in the body. Brown fat is a remarkable sort of adipose tissue, dark in colour and with a more solid, glandular-like structure than ordinary fatty tissue. It is not present in all mammals, but it is generally better developed in hibernating than in non-hibernating species. The oxidation of brown fat is a major source of heat to the body. The rapid rewarming which occurs during arousals from hibernation must rely heavily upon this thermogenic source, although of course other heat producing mechanisms such as shivering are also brought into play. In the early part of arousal, blood flow is restricted to the anterior regions of the body, warming only the essential organs, and at the same time reducing heat loss. In some hibernators, brown fat also seems to act as a store for androgens, which could explain the sustained libido during, and precocious sexual activity after, hibernation in some mammals even though the testes are involuted.

The test drops into torpor before true hibernation in some mammals were at one time thought to indicate 'acclimatization' to reduced temperatures. But test drops are by no means universal in hibernating mammals. In fact, skipped heart beats, followed by slowing of the heart and a reduction in metabolic rate which is accompanied by a reduction in body temperature, signals the entrance into hibernation of many mammals. The lower heart rate of hibernating animals is not associated with a markedly reduced blood pressure, which remains relatively high. Again, vascular tone is maintained during hibernation, and in some species peripheral resistance is increased as the animals enter hibernation.

The reduced temperatures of the body of a hibernating animal does not indicate the complete lack of temperature control which operates normally in summer and in non-hibernators. At ambient temperatures between 5 and 15°C, the hibernator maintains a body temperature about 1°C above that of its surroundings. Moreover, if the environmental temperature falls to potentially lethal values, arousal quickly follows. Thus the temperature regulating mechanism operates as efficiently for survival during hibernation as it does during the higher temperatures of summer. Hibernating mammals cannot be considered to be 'primitive' homeotherms, unable to regulate their body temperatures during the winter cold: they are in one sense more advanced homeotherms with a 'thermostat' which can be set at different levels inside and outside hibernation.

The sustained function of the temperature regulator during the low temperatures of hibernation is perhaps the single most important difference between hibernating and non-hibernating species. Although there must be concomitant adaptive changes at the cellular level in nerves and muscle (including the heart) to withstand prolonged periods at low temperatures, these can be found also in non-hibernating arctic residents, particularly at the body extremities. But the maintenance of physiological control during hibernation differentiates uniquely the hibernator from other non-hibernating mammals which have been made hypothermic. This implies that the fundamental mechanisms controlling hibernation are to be found in the central and sympathetic nervous systems.

Arousal from hibernation can be induced by high or low temperatures and by physical disturbances involving touch and pressure. Spontaneous arousals can also occur, perhaps because essential metabolic precursors have become exhausted, or because waste products require elimination. Whatever the reason for such arousals, the fact that they happen supports the hypothesis of sustained integrated physiological control during the low temperatures of hibernation.

Mammalian hibernation, with immediate control centred upon the nervous system, is basically different from insect diapause, where immediate control is exercised by the endocrine system. Although the final control system takes different paths in the mammals and the insects, both groups make use of nervous integration and co-ordination to appreciate and respond to environmental tokens with the ultimate goal of dormancy. It is perhaps to be expected that the more highly organized mammals retain a much closer individual control of dormancy than is experienced in the developmental arrests of insects.

Mammalian dormancy has a great deal in common with bird migration. In both birds and mammals, the responses are designed to avoid unfavourable seasons. The control mechanisms for both hibernation and migration are centred in the nervous system. Preparations for both migration and hibernation, including the storage of food reserves and the involution of endocrine tissues, are similar in both groups of animals and are dependent upon environmental tokens, especially photoperiod. The final stimulus which evokes the particular response is different in the two groups—predominantly photoperiod for migration, and temperature for hibernation. That birds have found migration to be more advantageous than hibernation is undoubtedly due to their far greater mobility compared with mammals. Even so, the particular avoidance mechanisms are not confined exclusively to each group: some mammals do migrate, and at least one bird is known, the Poor-Will of California (*Phalaenoptilus nuttallii*), which hibernates!

Chapter 10
Animal Colours

Some animals, for example many plankton, coelenterates, some scyphozoans, a few pelagic gastropods and some fishes, are almost devoid of colour and therefore to varying degrees are translucent. It follows that such animals are, as a result, less conspicuous. On the other hand, pigments are found in all groups of animals from the protozoa through to the higher mammals. They are put to a variety of uses, for example, in visual systems, for the transportation and storage of oxygen and also, of course, to provide colour to the body covering. Pigments used in general body coloration are extremely varied in their chemical nature. Carotenoids and melanins are of very common occurrence, whereas other pigments such as pteridines, ommochromes, quinones and flavins are found only in a few groups of animals. We can classify animal colours into two major categories; one in which the colour is formed by pigments present within the epidermal cells or underlying tissues and the others in which colour is formed as a result of the physical properties of the skin. Colours of this latter category are called structural colours and are caused by physical phenomena such as interference, diffraction, scattering and dispersal of the light falling on the animal. Iridescent colours, that is those which change according to the angle from which the animal is viewed, are formed by interference or diffraction effects.

The variety of animal colours is prodigious and animals are coloured differently for particular reasons. Many animals are coloured brightly and possess colour patterns which render them especially conspicuous. Such patterns provide important recognition marks. For example, they may warn potential predators that the animal possesses defence mechanisms, or be poisonous or extremely distasteful. In addition, there are many harmless animals with conspicuous warning colours, but their advertisement is false for they depend on the reputation of harmful species. In many other instances the colour of animals tends to harmonize with that of their immediate environment. Such protective or cryptic coloration ensures that the animal is less subject to predation. There have been many successful experiments which have quantified and verified the obvious selective advantage of protective coloration. One, perhaps now classical, demonstration of the importance of protective coloration is the work of Kettlewell, on industrial mellanization. He demonstrated a clear selective advantage for the dark-coloured phenotype of the moth, *Biston betularia*, in polluted or industrial areas. The light-coloured phenotype is more conspicuous in such areas and is subjected to greater predation. As we shall see later in this section, there are many animals who are able to change reversibly their colour or colour patterns. These reversible changes may enable them to merge with their immediate background or can make the animal more obvious. In animals which change colour to merge with their background, it seems a plausible hypothesis that they do so to increase their chances of survival. Cryptic coloration is, of course, advantageous to prey to reduce the possibility of discovery by predators and of benefit also to themselves in that they hide their presence from potential prey. It is unfortunate that whereas animals which are constant in their protective coloration have been proved clearly to be at an advantage, this is not obvious in animals which undergo rapid and reversible colour change.

The significance of colour change in some animals has been disputed and indeed many animals may change colour to facilitate thermoregulation. Lizards, such as *Phrynosoma* which live in the desert are light in colour at high temperatures to reduce heat uptake and facilitate radiation of heat. At low temperatures the lizard darkens to facilitate heat uptake. Such mechanisms are of utmost importance as part of the complicated repertoire of physiological and behavioural responses which cold blooded animals possess to maintain their body temperature at acceptable levels. It has been suggested also that changes in pigment distribution are important in protecting internal body organs from intense illumination. In other animals, marked colour changes occur which are related to seasonal mating activity. More rapid colour changes can occur in lizards and cephalopods during mating behaviour.

Colour change may be restricted to the sudden exposure of brightly coloured areas of the animal or it may be a much more complicated process involving a number of organs and cellular events to alter the amount of pigment exposed. There are two forms of this latter type of colour change. One is concerned with slow long-term changes, morphological colour change, and the other with short-term rapid changes in colour, physiological colour change.

Morphological colour change

Most multi-celled animals have characteristic colour patterns, which often may be static, or change only slowly during growth and development or during sexual maturation. In some instances morphological colour change is concerned with seasonal changes as in the production of winter plumage. Morphological colour change depends upon the formation and destruction of pigment.

Physiological colour change

Physiological colour change involves the rapid alteration of the distribution of pigment within the integument. The pigments in such instances are contained within specialized effector organs called chromatophores. The range of animals which are able to rapidly change their colour in this way is rather restricted. In the invertebrates a greater variety of groups exhibit physiological colour change, but only the cephalopod molluscs (cuttlefish, octopuses and squids) and the crustacea contain many species which change colour habitually.

There are two types of chromatophore, one type restricted to the cephalopod molluscs and the other form is present in all other animals showing physiological colour change. Cephalopod chromatophores consist of a small sac containing pigment granules; attached to the sac wall is a stellate array of radial muscle fibres. The sac wall is elastic and when the muscle fibres contract or relax the shape of the pigment mass is altered and thus changes in the colour of the animal are produced (Fig. 10.1).

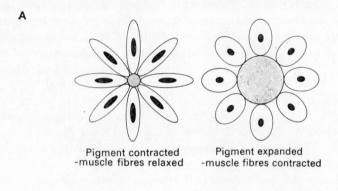

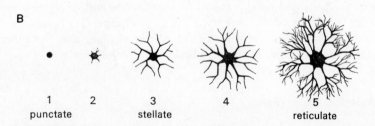

Figure 10.1. (A) Diagrams showing pigment expansion and contraction in cephalopod chromatophores. (B) The Chromatophore Index. An arbitrary scale used to quantify the degree of dispersion or contraction of pigment in non-molluscan chromatophores.

The other type of chromatophore of more universal occurrence consists of an irregularly branched cell. Pigment movement is caused by the cytoplasm of the cell and is not dependent upon contractile elements (Fig. 10.1B). By using the Chromatophore Index shown in Fig. 10.1B, quantitative estimates can be made of the degree of dispersion or contraction of the pigment. Unlike molluscan chromatophores, the chromatophores of other animals do not change their shape. The exact mechanisms by which the distribution of the pigment is altered is still disputed. Many workers have implicated the state of the protoplasm in the movement of pigment within the cell. The dispersed state is associated with the sol state and as the protoplasm becomes more viscous the pigment granules clump together. Other workers have coupled changes in the state of the protoplasm with contractile elements present within the cells. However, more recent research suggests that pigment movement depends upon electropotential gradients within the cells and negatively charged pigment granules. Ionic changes are involved also, K^+ causes clumping, while Na^+ has the reverse effect. Indeed some hormones such as melanophore stimulating hormone (MSH) which disperse melanin granules are only able to exert their effect if Na^+ is present. The analysis of membrane permeability and trans-membrane potentials seems likely to provide the explanations of pigment movement.

Not all animals which undergo physiological colour change do so by dispersal or concentration of pigment within chromatophores. Some beetles exhibit reversible changes in colour but do not possess chromatophores. Their colours depend on the physical phenomenon of disruption in the light reflected from the elytra. In tortoise beetles (*Cassida* and allies) hydration and dehydration of the elytra changes markedly their iridescent colours by altering the thickness of the interference layers. The giant beetle (*Dynastes*) can bring about also reversible changes in colour (between yellow and black) of its elytra by changing the state of hydration of the cuticle. The cuticle of the elytra consists of three layers, an outer transparent layer, a yellowish spongy middle layer and a black basal layer. When the yellow middle layer is air-filled it is optically heterogeneous and reflects yellow light. However, when this yellow layer is fluid-filled it is optically homogeneous, light passes through it and is absorbed by the black layer below and the elytra appear black. The elytra can begin to change colour from black to yellow within 30 sec to 2 min of a change in hydration.

There are only a few invertebrates which possess a marked ability to change their colour patterns by rapidly altering the distribution of the pigment present in the chromatophores. The groups which best exhibit physiological colour change are the cephalopod molluscs and a number of groups of crustacea; in both instances the chromatophores are under a central control. In the cephalopods the distribution of pigment within the chromatophores is solely under nervous control. The colour of the environment or changes in it are perceived through the eyes and this sensory input is relayed to the chromatophores *via* the nervous system. The pigment distribution is altered by the contraction and relaxation of muscles attached to it. Since the control of the chromatophores in cephalopods involves a neuro-muscular mechanism, total colour change can occur in less than a second.

In squids the chromatophores are in three layers, bright yellow near the surface, a middle layer of orange red and the deepest layer is of brown chromatophores. Other colours may be present from green and blue structural colours. In a swimming *Sepia* the outline of the animal is broken by a 'zebra' effect of dark transverse stripes. Over sandy areas 'the colour can be quickly changed to a mottled brown and grey, while over a white background the chromatophores fully contract to produce total pallor. Indeed the repertoire of colour change is so diverse that the squid can to a recognizable extent merge with a black and white chequered surface! As well as possessing this marked cryptic behaviour the squid is also on other occasions able to exhibit vivid changes in colour. This adoption of a conspicuous appearance is probably an attempt to frighten off intruders.

In the crustacea the chromatophores are not innervated and are controlled entirely by hormones. Shrimps and prawns are capable of spectacular changes in colour and such changes have been of interest to biologists since the time of Aristotle, but it was not until 1928 that the blood of shrimps and prawns was shown to contain a substance which affected the movement of pigment within the chromatophores. This discovery of a blood borne factor stimulating an effector organ (the chromatophore) was the first indisputable evidence for the presence of hormones in invertebrates. Systematic examination of the body tissues revealed that the eyestalks were potent sources of chromactivating hormones. The sinus gland in the eyestalk, although comprising only 1/100 the volume of the eyestalk, was found to contain more than 80% of the hormonal activity. Once the concept of neurosecretion (see pp. 124, 143) was established it was realized that the chromactivating substances of the sinus gland were produced by the X-organ neurosecretory cells and stored in the sinus gland prior to release into the blood. Other neurosecretory chromactivating substances were soon discovered in the central nervous system (CNS) outside the eyestalk in the circum-oesophageal connectives and the post-oesophageal connectives (Fig. 10.2).

The pigment granules in crustacean chromatophores, in general with those of other animals, respond directly to light but we shall concentrate upon the regulatory mechanisms which the animal employs to control pigment dispersion. It was quickly realized that the chromatophores responded to more than one hormone. In the common shrimp (*Crangon*) the black pigment is controlled by hormones released from both the post-commissural organs and the eyestalks. A peptide hormone from the commissural organs concentrates the black pigment and causes the body of the shrimp to show an overall whitening; a protein hormone extracted from the same post-commissural organs acts in exactly the opposite way and disperses pigment in the black chromatophores of both the body and tail and in consequence makes the animal dark overall. The eyestalks also contain two hormones which act upon the black pigment, one causes concentration in the body chromatophores and the other hormone concentrates the black pigment in both the body and tail. The four hormones (Fig. 10.2) act differentially to produce a particular dispersion pattern of the pigment. A particular chromatophore state is caused by a balance between antagonistically acting hormones. The hormones either cause expansion or contraction of the pigment, but in their absence the pigment does not revert to its opposite state. When caused to expand by one hormone the pigment can only be made to contract by the action of a second hormone; removal of the hormone causing expansion does not in itself produce contraction. This description of the hormonal regulation of the black chromatophores outlines the principles involved in the regulation of the dispersion and contraction of pigment in other chromatophores and in many other crustacea. The rapid change from full expansion to full contraction is possible because of the antagonistic action of the hormones and the change is most efficient when a large amount of one hormone occurs when the concentration of its antagonist is falling.

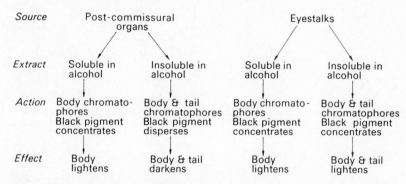

Source	Post-commissural organs		Eyestalks	
Extract	Soluble in alcohol	Insoluble in alcohol	Soluble in alcohol	Insoluble in alcohol
Action	Body chromatophores Black pigment concentrates	Body & tail chromatophores Black pigment disperses	Body chromatophores Black pigment concentrates	Body & tail chromatophores Black pigment concentrates
Effect	Body lightens	Body & tail darkens	Body lightens	Body & tail lightens

Figure 10.2. Control of the dispersion of the black pigment within the chromatophores of the shrimp (*Crangon*) Extraction of the eyestalk or post-commissural organs with alcohol or water reveals the presence of four different hormones involved in this control.

The control of pigment dispersion is by hormones carried in the blood, but how is the release of the regulatory hormones co-ordinated and geared to changes in the background coloration of the environment? Since the chromatophores are of considerable importance for protective coloration it is not surprising that both direct and reflected light control the colour of the animal. The different illumination has an effect upon sensory units, in particular regions of the eyes. These sensory impulses act through the CNS to regulate the release of the dispersing and concentrating hormones. It is probable that the stimuli from the different regions of the eyes are co-ordinated and integrated at special centres in the CNS. It is the signals from these integration centres which bring about the release of the appropriate hormones. Figure 10.3 shows the effects of differential illumination of the eye upon the dispersion of pigment in the melanophores (chromatophores containing only black pigment) of the sea slater, *Ligia*. When placed on a dark background with the dorsal region of the eye illuminated (as would happen under natural conditions with direct light upon a dark substrate) the pigment is fully dispersed (Melanophore index 4·7) and the animal tones in with its background. If illumination is on the ventral surface or from all directions, as would happen with direct light and light reflected from a light background, the pigment is concentrated as the animal attempts to tone in with its light background.

In the vertebrates the ability to show physiological colour change is restricted to cold blooded forms such as fish, amphibia and reptiles. Some vertebrates exert a dual control over the movement of pigment in their chromatophores; utilizing both nervous and hormonal control mechanisms. In the amphibia,

A   The method of illuminating different parts of the eye of the sea slater, *Ligia*.

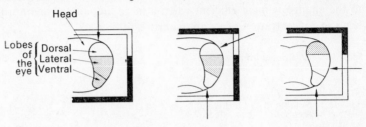

B   The state of the melanophores in *Ligia* when different parts of the eyes are illuminated.

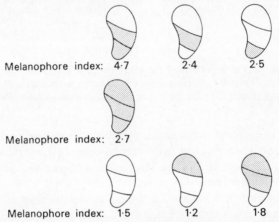

Figure 10.3. Effects of illuminating different parts of the compound eyes upon the state of the chromatophores in *Ligia*. (A) Method used to illuminate different parts of the eye. (B) Relationship between illumination and the Chromatophore Index. When the dorsal part of the eye is illuminated, as would happen naturally with direct light upon a dark background, the chromatophore pigment disperses fully, darkening the animal to tone with its surroundings. When the eye is illuminated from the ventral surface, or from several directions, as would happen with direct light together with light reflected from the background, the chromatophore pigment concentrates, toning the animal with a light background. (From K. C. Highnam and L. Hill (1969). *The comparative endocrinology of the invertebrates*. Edward Arnold.)

however, the control is purely hormonal and there is no direct innervation of the chromatophores. Amphibia are varied in their colour, but normally it is only the movement of the pigment in the melanophores which is responsible for the pronounced colour changes. The melanophores lie deepest in the skin and are overlaid with cells containing other pigments. The movement of pigment in the melanophores is controlled by hormones released from the pituitary gland. It has been known since 1916 that tadpoles deprived of their pituitaries remained permanently pale. This observation suggested strongly that the pituitary could be the source of a hormone which brought about dispersion of the melanin. More detailed studies of chromatophore control in *Rana* and *Xenopus* have suggested that two hormones from the pituitary may be involved. The most fully understood effects are those of the MSH. This hormone, produced by the pars intermedia (middle lobe) of the pituitary causes the pigment in the melano-phores to expand. Under its influence frogs become very dark but it is also of interest that MSH will produce darkening in mammals and fishes as well. From detailed studies of changes in the Chromatophore Index when frogs are changed from a white to a black background and *vice versa*, the existence of a melanocyte concentrating hormone released from the pituitary has been postulated. The two hormones are antagonistic in their actions (this of course is very similar to the control of the melanophores in crustacea). Stimulation of the peripheral retinal elements seems to cause release of the concentrating hormone, whereas MSH is released following illumination of the basal elements. Thus, in an illuminated environment, MSH is always released into the blood, the responses of frogs to dark and light backgrounds depends upon the concentrating hormone secreted into the blood. The final colour of the frog in response to the background coloration, depends upon the relative amounts of the two hormones present in the blood. Direct evidence for the existence of concentrating hormone has come from examining the responses of frogs to environmental stimuli after the frogs have been subjected to a variety of operations interfering with the normal func-tioning of the pituitary. This approach to the analysis of chromatophore function is a very good example of the benefit of detailed studies of intact ani-mals in their natural or near natural environments, but also importantly a full understanding only comes from a combination of this type of study with knowledge gained from experiments involving interference with the animals' endocrine system.

If the anterior lobe of the pituitary is removed, frogs respond normally to changes in their background but if the pars tuberalis is removed at the same time they are no longer able to respond to background changes and the pigment in the melanophores is maximally dispersed. However, when the posterior lobe is removed (this operation also removes the pars intermedia) the animals are maximally pale, but removal of the whole gland leaves the animal in a non-responsive state with the pigment slightly dispersed. Obviously a concentrating hormone could be present in the pars tuberalis and MSH present in the inter-mediate lobe or posterior lobe. Further support for the existence of two factors controlling dispersion of melanin comes from comparisons of the effects of injection of pituitary extract into normal animals, animals with the whole of the pituitary removed and those with only the posterior lobe removed (Fig. 10.4). If the posterior lobe is present, more hormone is needed to produce a given response than in completely hypophysectomized animals. This phenomenon is best explained by the presence of an antagonist in intact animals or in those in which the pars tuberalis remains. This concentrating factor is of course missing in those animals from which all the pituitary has been removed.

In fishes, colour changes in response to changes in background also depend upon visual stimulation. The regulatory pathways involve not only endocrine glands and blood borne hormones, but also efferent nervous pathways which

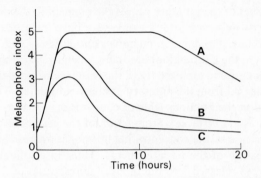

Figure 10.4. The effect of injection of pituitary extracts (containing MSH) upon the melanophores of the toad, *Xenopus*. The animals were kept on a white background. A = whole pituitary removed; B = intact control; C = post lobe of pituitary removed. Each group were injected with the same amount of extract at time 0.

directly innervate the chromatophores—the chemical mediators affecting the chromatophores are released at the nerve terminals. Fishes show, however, a considerable variety in the mechanisms involved in control of their chromatophores. They can be classified into three main groups differing from each other in the extent to which their chromatophores are innervated. Some fish possess chromatophores which are doubly innervated, one fibre for dispersal and a separate one for bringing about concentration of the pigment. Other fish possess only a single innervation of their chromatophores and this is always responsible for concentrating the pigment. In the remaining group the chromatophores are regulated solely by blood borne factors.

Most teleosts possess doubly innervated chromatophores. The action of the concentrating fibre is readily shown when a ganglion of the CNS is electrically stimulated; the area of skin innervated by this ganglion shows blanching. If this area of skin is denervated, stimulation of the ganglion no longer produces a blanching effect. However, stimulation of an adjacent ganglion will produce blanching in an adjacent area of skin. Obviously blanching is due to localized responses at nerve terminals with different areas of skin being controlled by different regions of the CNS. No substances which are freely diffusible in the blood are involved, concentration is produced by an adrenalin-like substance released at the nerve terminals and has a purely localized effect. The concentration is reversed either by breakdown of the stimulating substances by the chromatophore or the gradual diffusion of the chemical out of the chromatophores.

Figure 10.5 illustrates the evidence which suggests that fibres exist which are responsible for controlling dispersion of pigment. If the fish *Fundulus* is kept on an illuminated white background, the pigment is of course concentrated, but

Fundulus tail

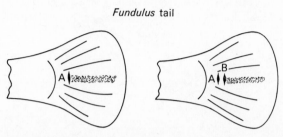

Figure 10.5. Diagrams showing the effect of a section of the caudal nerves upon pigment dispersion in the fish *Fundulus* kept on an illuminated white background. Following cut A the pigment disperses temporarily and a dark band is formed. A few days later a further cut B also produces transient darkening. The reasons are obscure.

if some of the caudal nerves are cut a band of the fin which was innervated by these sectioned nerves darkens quickly and takes surprisingly a few days to fade. If a second cut is made nearer to the extremity of the tail (as in Fig. 10.5B) the transient darkening effect will reappear. However, in spite of the considerable researches which have been carried out into colour change in teleosts, this phenomenon of dispersion is imperfectly understood. The effects of the first nerve section could be explained by transection of concentrating fibres; the effects of the second cut can only be explained by the restimulation of the dispersing nerve fibres, which were transected and stimulated by the first cut. The evidence does suggest a double innervation even though it is somewhat unsatisfactory. The dispersing agent is thought to be acetylcholine.

In many fishes such as cyclostomes and elasmobranchs the sole control of the chromatophores is by hormones. Blood-borne factors are also of importance in other fish. In the eel *Anguilla* colour change is under hormonal control predominantly but other factors are also involved. The complexity of chromatophore regulation in fish is illustrated in Fig. 10.6.

It seems likely that humoral control of chromatophores is a primitive phenomenon and during evolution an element of nervous control has been superimposed. The development of a direct nervous control does of course allow a more rapid response of the animal's colour to match changes in background.

The ability of chameleons to change colour is well known. The chromatophores in these animals are under the control of the sympathetic nervous system. In other reptiles such as the iguanid lizards chromatophore control is by humoral factors.

Chromactivating hormones are produced by endocrine glands other than the pituitary. Adrenalin and nor-adrenalin have often marked concentrating effects upon melanophores. Another catecholamine which exerts a pronounced effect

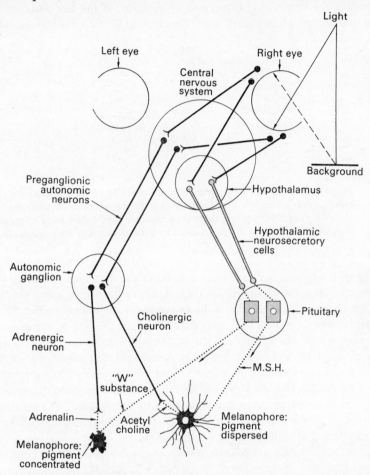

Figure 10.6. Control of the melanophores of the eel *Anguilla* based on the observations of Waring (1940) and Parker (1943). Only pathways originating in one eye are indicated. (From E. Scharrer and B. Scharrer (1963) *Neuroendocrinology*, Columbia University Press.)

upon melanophores is melatonin (N-acetyl-5-methoxy tryptamine) which is 100,000-fold more potent than nor-adrenalin in concentrating the melanin in frog's skin. Melatonin is found in the pineal body and it seems very likely that the pineal is involved also in colour responses but as yet in an ill-defined manner.

Chapter 11
Biotic Interactions

For any population, the 'total environment' may be defined as a combination of the purely physical or abiotic *milieu* (geographical features, prevailing physico-chemical and climatic conditions and terrain) and the organic or biotic *milieu* (all the other local populations of plants and animals in that region, including competitors, predators, parasites). Their influence on populations, and the relative importance of these two components of the environment are covered in the standard ecological texts. However, for any individual member of a population, the biotic environment will also include other members of the same population. It is important to realize that while organisms are capable of receiving signals from their environment, they are also capable of emitting them. The importance of this aspect of the biotic environment has received little attention until recently.

Just as cells within a tissue (a cell population) may interact with each other (pp. 24–26), individuals of a population may experience mutual interactions. Examples of such interactions are too numerous for a comprehensive account to be given here. Audio and visual signals, while clearly being important in some species, cannot be dealt with in an account of this length. Similarly, it will not be possible to include a full treatment of chemically mediated interspecific interactions between hosts and their parasites, and predators and their prey. Only some examples of behavioural and chemical intraspecific interactions, i.e. between animals of the same species will be discussed. Some interspecific interactions between animals and their food materials will be included, since chemical signals produced by plants appear to be an important component of the biotic environment of some herbivores.

Aggregations and gregariousness in animals

In nature, many animal species, at some time in their life history, are found to be gregariously distributed. It is the causes and effects of this gregariousness that are of particular interest. Many of these animals possess either spontaneous, or chemically-mediated, behavioural mechanisms (or a combination of both) which bring about and maintain the spatial organization and distribution of the population; similar mechanisms exist in uniformly dispersed animals. Chemical messengers or pheromones which are substances released by one animal to affect the behaviour of another are known to be produced by a wide variety of animals. They may be employed to release fixed behavioural patterns (releaser pheromones), or to influence the metabolism or physiology of the receptor individuals, which may indirectly affect subsequent behaviour (primer pheromones). Some pheromones act in both ways. Among the lower animals, such diverse forms as cellular slime moulds, barnacles, and bark beetles, all provide examples of aggregations which are brought about by releaser pheromones.

Cellular slime moulds

The active feeding stage of cellular slime moulds, such as *Dictyostelium*, consists of free-living amoebae. These single, unicellular, non-ciliated amoebae feed on bacteria. They grow, divide and glide about independently of other amoebae until the population reaches its maximum density, i.e. when growth and division are slowing down as the bacterial food supply becomes depleted. At this time, groups of amoebae stream towards central collection points and form large single masses at each centre. Each large mass (10^3 to 2×10^5 single amoebae) becomes vertically elongated and covered by a sheath secreted by the constituent cells. These masses, or pseudo-plasmodia, bend over and begin to migrate in a horizontal plane. When migration ceases, the pseudo-plasmodia assume a vertical position again and differentiate to form a stalk which bears an apical spore mass. Spores liberated and dispersed from this structure each hatch to give a single amoeba which is capable of initiating a whole new cycle.

It has been known for many years that the aggregation process is initiated by a chemical substance, acrasin, which is produced by the individual amoebae. A second product of these cells is an extracellular enzyme, acrasinase, which destroys acrasin. Acrasinase is thought to be of importance in maintaining steep concentration gradients of acrasin. Recently, acrasin has been tentatively identified as cyclic-3,5-adenosine monophosphate (cyclic-3,5-AMP), and acrasinase as a phosphodiesterase (which specifically converts cyclic-3,5-AMP to 5-AMP, thus inactivating it). Both cyclic-3,5-AMP and phosphodiesterase are synthesized and released into the external medium by *Dictyostelium*.

Acrasinase is produced at all times, even before aggregation, but it is not yet known whether the volume of production varies with time. Acrasin is produced only during aggregation when the individual amoebae become very sensitive to acrasin (or externally applied cyclic-3,5-AMP). If all the amoebae start to produce acrasin (or become sensitive to it) synchronously, then this would not explain the observed aggregations. In order to break up the random pattern of distribution, the cells must differ in the timing of either their acrasin production or the development of their sensitivity. There is evidence that the cells at the end of the vegetative (growing and dividing) stage do differ in size and physiological state, and it is assumed that the time of onset of acrasin production or increased sensitivity will vary among the cells. Since aggregation coincides with the cessation of growth, perhaps the few cells that inevitably cease growing and dividing ahead of the majority, may be the first cells to form aggregation centres. If this is so, these few cells, scattered here and there, could cause a discontinuity in the even distribution of amoebae in one of two ways; if one cell produced more acrasin than its neighbours it would attract the surrounding cells, or, if one cell became prematurely sensitive to acrasin, it would move towards neighbouring cells. It is not known which of these possibilities is correct or, indeed, whether acrasin production and increased sensitivity can be separated. In non-aggregating mutants, both acrasin production and sensitivity are lacking and it may be that the two processes are in some way linked at the biochemical level.

Many unresolved problems exist in our understanding of the mechanism by which cellular slime moulds aggregate, but the identification of cyclic-3,5-AMP as an acrasin is of importance. This substance is an internal product of many animal cells and appears to be involved in the action of some vertebrate and invertebrate hormones. J. B. S. Haldane has suggested that communication among protozoan cells must have preceded the formation of metazoans and that this communication was probably chemical. The employment of an existing cellular metabolite as a pheromone would seem a reasonable possibility from an evolutionary viewpoint.

Settlement factors and attractants

It is now accepted generally that the larvae of many sessile marine organisms do not settle at random, but often exercise a choice of habitat in that metamorphosis may be delayed until suitable conditions are found. Adult barnacles are found distributed gregariously and chemical signals have been shown to be important in the settling behaviour of their larvae. In *Balanus*, the chemical involved, a non-dialysable, heat stable, proteinaceous substance, is not an attractant as such. Its presence will promote settlement, sometimes even on substances that normally would not be chosen by the larvae. No evidence of chemotaxis is found; several substrates may be investigated by any individual larva which responds to the factor only after alighting on the treated surface.

Substances promoting settlement in *Balanus* larvae are found in extracts of many species of barnacles and other arthropods, but the most active factor is obtained from extracts made from adult *Balanus*. There is, therefore, some degree of specificity in the chemical involved, and the presence of the settling factor (derived from adults) on a substrate previously colonized by barnacles, will explain the gregarious settling behaviour of barnacle larvae. Settlement factors have been described for larvae of other marine organisms, such as, for example, sea anemones, and sedentary polychaetes; they appear to act in a

will be further developed in the following discussion of locust and aphid populations.

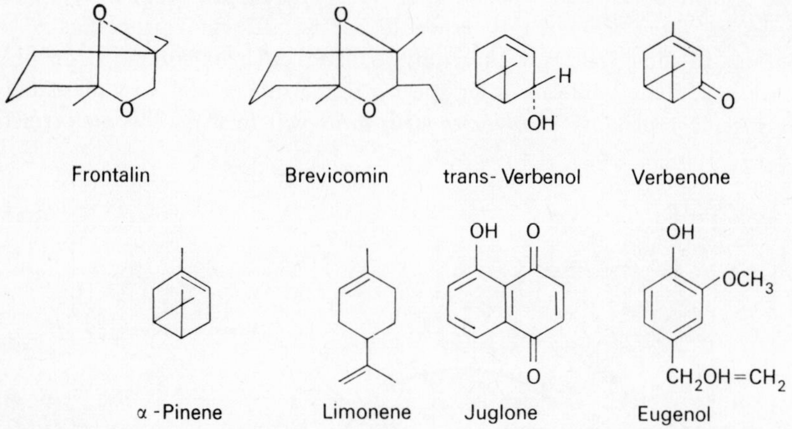

| Frontalin | Brevicomin | trans- Verbenol | Verbenone |

| α -Pinene | Limonene | Juglone | Eugenol |

Figure 11.2. The structure of some important chemicals in the biotic environment of the insects discussed in Chapter 11.

Density dependent phenomena

There are many examples of gregariousness in animals which, at high population densities, may eventually result in profound physiological and behavioural changes within individuals of the population. Such density dependent changes may include growth inhibition, reduced fecundity and dispersal. In most cases, behavioural mechanisms operate to maintain the gregariousness of the individuals, even at high densities, thus increasing the effective population density. Pheromones may be involved in establishing gregariousness as in the examples that we have already discussed and also in mediating density dependent physiological changes.

LOCUSTS

Locusts differ from grasshoppers in possessing a swarming or dispersive phase. The extreme dispersive phase, *gregaria*, and the extreme non-swarming phase, *solitaria*, differ in appearance to such an extent that until Sir Boris Uvarov put forward his now famous theory in 1921, it was not realized that the three species then known as *Locusta migratoria*, *L. danica* and *L. migratorioides* were actually forms of a single continuously polymorphic stock. Solitarious and gregarious locusts differ in many ways; the most striking, but perhaps not the most significant, being differences in pigmentation. Solitarious locusts tend to be green, grey or drab, whereas gregarious locusts are usually conspicuously coloured, with a yellowish or orange background marked boldly and striped with black. Perhaps the most important difference between the phases is in their behaviour. As their names suggest, solitarious locusts tend to ignore their fellows whereas the gregarious forms are intensely sociable; they seek and maintain the closest contact with their companions.

What is the relationship between the phases of locusts? It is clear from laboratory experiments that crowding solitarious locusts, or isolating gregarious locusts, can initiate a reversal of the original phase characters. Some changes brought about in this way may occur rapidly (within weeks for pigmentation changes) but others may take longer (generations for morphometric changes). Phase changes appear to be brought about by an increase or decrease in the total sensory input from the environment to the locust. Crowding, with its consequent increase in mutual sensory stimulation, will induce or maintain a shift towards gregariousness, whereas isolation, a reduction in sensory input, favours solitariousness. Crowding or isolating locusts in the laboratory does not produce such extreme examples of *gregaria* or *solitaria* as are found in the field. It is evident that other environmental factors, along with population density, are important in phase determination.

In insects, it is well established that environmental cues may influence neuro-endocrine activity and many workers have therefore attempted to relate phase differences to changes in endocrine activity. Briefly, it is thought that solitarious individuals differ from the gregarious forms in having more active corpora allata and prothoracic glands. It is suggested also that the phases may differ in the activity of the cerebral neurosecretory cells. However, the evidence for hormonal involvement in the determination of all but a few phase characteristics is inconclusive. Whilst locust phases may differ in certain characteristics, the solitarious and gregarious forms share many essential physiological and metabolic functions which are known to be under the control of neuro-endocrine factors. It is therefore difficult to accept that phase determination is due simply to gross differences in the titres of the established insect hormones and it is most likely that a combination of nervous, hormonal and genetic factors is involved.

The ecological significance of locust polymorphism is not as clear as may appear at first sight. The phase theory, as it was first proposed, envisaged that solitarious locusts occupy a fixed habitat which includes the so-called outbreak area. Under favourable conditions the resident solitarious population undergoes a tremendous increase which may lead, especially when local crowding around areas of suitable vegetation takes place, to the formation of gregarious individuals whose natural behavioural characteristics will reinforce this crowding by deliberate aggregation. Emigration follows under suitable conditions; vast numbers of locusts take off in a sustained emigration flight which is frequently downwind. Swarming therefore relieves the congestion in the outbreak area and the remaining population reverts to the *solitaria* phase. Meanwhile, the swarming *gregaria* finally descend and breed. The new generation of voracious locusts causes great damage to crops and other vegetation but often, before the end

evidence in support of this theory is accumulating for some species, it is realized now that interactions between the aphids themselves play an important, if not dominant, part in the production of winged adults.

Early investigations concerning the role of the host plant in the determination of wing dimorphism, failed often to take into account the possibility of aphid-aphid interactions. Similarly, experiments on crowding were subject to the criticism that food could be a limiting factor in crowded populations. Recently, however, more carefully controlled and critical experiments have shown conclusively that both crowding and nutrition are important in the determination of winged forms.

In the sycamore aphid (*Drepanosiphum platinoides*), the initial colonization of the host tree involves a non-random settling in which some leaves, or parts of leaves, are avoided completely. The aphids form loose groups occupying restricted parts of the leaf surface and they settle preferentially where they can just touch one or more of their fellows with their antennae. Laboratory experiments with two strains of the pea aphid (*Acyrthosiphon pisum*) have shown that in the pink strain, an initial meeting of two aphids is followed by a rapid withdrawal of one or other of the aphids once contact has been made between the antennae of one and the legs of the other. This may not prevent further contact but excessive contact is avoided wherever possible. The green strain of the pea aphid, however, reacts in a very less intense manner and contact between aphids is not avoided to the same extent as in the pink strain. It is perhaps hardly surprising that the pink form is exceptionally sensitive to crowding (producing many winged individuals) whereas the green strain is relatively insensitive.

The response to crowding appears to be due to tactile stimulation alone and removal of the antennae which bear numerous thick-walled bristles, thought to be mechanoreceptors, diminishes the crowding response considerably in some species. However, tactile bristles on the legs and the body may act also as mechanoreceptors; a possibility which would explain why removal of the antennae does not abolish completely the crowding response. In some species, stimulation of these tactile bristles on the legs and body may be more important than the antennal receptors in initiating the production of winged forms in response to the crowding stimulus.

Sensitivity to crowding varies with the stage of development and with the species. In some species crowding of the parents is the decisive factor, while in others, the period of sensitivity may be post-natal; in others a combination of both conditions may exist. However, in some species a brief period of crowding of adults will induce the production of winged forms in the first batch of larvae. This suggests that determination may occur shortly before birth and that the mother in some way influences the fate of the developing embryo. Similarly, crowding of the third or fourth instar larvae of some species will cause them, when adults (even after two moults), to produce winged progeny. The crowding stimulus is therefore in some way 'remembered' until just before parturition, when determination occurs. Clearly, while the causal factors are known in part, the mechanisms involved in the determination of winged forms are likely to be very complicated.

The environmental control of the differentiation of non-winged and winged morphs, undoubtedly acts through the insect's neuro-endocrine system. In insects, the corpora allata produce juvenile hormone, which is responsible for the expression of juvenile characters; its absence at a moult results in the replacement of juvenile by adult characters. In the majority of insects, the wings appear (as functional units) only at the larval/adult or pupal/adult moult and may, therefore, be regarded as adult characteristics. Usually non-winged aphids are considered as being more juvenile than their corresponding winged forms; an opinion which implies the involvement of juvenile hormone. Recent work has shown that wing formation can be diminished or suppressed by the application of juvenile hormone (or some of the substances which mimic its action) to developing, potential winged aphids. It has been suggested that if wing dimorphism is regulated by the concentration of juvenile hormone in the haemolymph, then developing larvae which are destined to become wingless adults should contain a large quantity of juvenile hormone. Such aphids show no obvious response to the application of additional juvenile hormone and this would appear to support this argument, although it should be emphasized that the endocrine control of polymorphism is not well understood.

The nature of the host plant may influence the normal response of aphids to a crowding stimulus and also may affect wing dimorphism directly. In the pea aphid, few winged individuals are produced by females reared singly on young leaves but when such females are transferred without crowding to mature leaves, they produce winged daughters after three days and similar responses have been shown for some other, but not all, aphid species. Aphids reared on seedlings show a lesser response to crowding than those on young plants but those fed on mature leaves show an enhanced response. In the latter case there is reason to suspect that it may not be a simple cumulative effect of two stimuli. Uncrowded aphids reared on seedlings and transferred to mature leaves will produce winged forms after three days, with the ultimate peak in the production of winged forms occurring a few days later. If the crowding stimulus is followed by a mature leaf stimulus, an immediate and intense production of winged forms follows which will always stay strong, long after the effect of the crowding stimulus would be expected to diminish. It seems, therefore, that some sort of synergistic interaction between the stimuli is possible.

What is the nature of the plant stimulus? The state of growth of the host plant will certainly affect the concentration of nutrients in the sap. Simple qualitative or quantitative differences in the constituents of the plant sap may be responsible for marked physiological changes in the aphids. However, it has been suggested that a simpler explanation is possible. Aphids become visibly restless on senescent vegetation and the numbers of encounters between aphids, and hence the crowding stimulus, would be greatly influenced by this behaviour. Although this may be a valid explanation for some species (although one may

and as a result, two major changes occur in the population; fecundity is reduced and mortality increases. The adaptation syndrome, as put forward by Selye, describes the endocrine responses which take place to enable the animal to maintain homeostasis under stress. Stress operates through the central nervous system to affect the hypothalamus and change the endocrine output of the pituitary

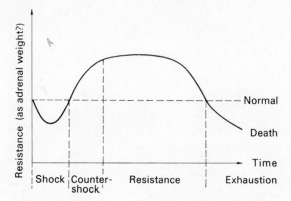

Figure 11.3. Changes in resistance to a specific stressor in different phases of the general adaptation syndrome.

gland (Fig. 11.4). In general, endocrine responses to stress act in such a way as to maintain the more essential homeostatic functions of the animal's physiology at the expense of other less important or less urgent requirements. In other words, as adequate supplies of oxygen to the tissues is maintained, blood glucose levels and Na^+ and K^+ balances are kept within normal limits and other physiological demands are met, while growth, reproduction and antibody production, for example, may be curtailed. If the stressful stimulus is short lived, the animal, having achieved a stage of resistance to the stimulus by virtue of the endocrine responses described above, recovers when the stressor is no longer present. If the stimulus persists, the resistance of the animal dwindles and death may follow due to the harmful side-effects of the very mechanisms which originally enabled the animal to survive. In particular, high concentrations of hormones from the adrenal cortex may have an eventual deleterious effect upon various target areas of the stress-adapted animal. Figure 11.4 outlines the endocrine adaptations envisaged in the social stress phenomenon.

There is much argument among ecologists and endocrinologists concerning this theory. First, there are reasonable grounds, which we need not elaborate at present, for questioning the validity of the endocrine mechanisms involved in the adaptation syndrome as envisaged by Selye. Second, and perhaps of more importance, there is very little direct evidence for the involvement of stress-mediated endocrine adaptation in wild mammalian populations.

Laboratory experiments have shown that, in rats and mice and a variety of field mammals, crowding will produce an increase in adrenal weight, and a decrease in the weights of the thymus and preputial glands. Adrenal hypertrophy is interpreted as indicating an increased production of adrenocortical hormones. Studies with some dense wild populations of the vole (*Microtus*) have shown that increased adrenal weight can be correlated with population density. However, most studies on crowded populations in nature have failed to find changes in

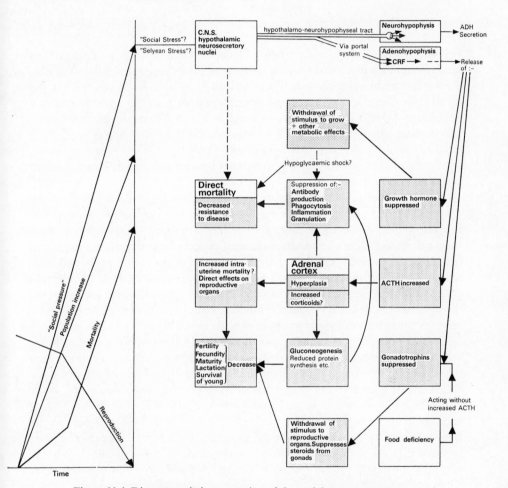

Figure 11.4. Diagrammatic interpretation of the social stress concept.

adrenal or gonadal weight. These observations are somewhat equivocable since adrenal weight need not be an accurate indication of adrenal activity; only when direct measurements of plasma corticosteroids and other hormones have been made will these questions be settled. Many authors, while accepting that social stress may operate in some wild mammalian populations, believe that it may be secondary to some other primary mechanism (food limitation, predation,

Chapter 12
The Impact of Man on the Environment

Animals and plants are interdependent, bound together in a series of associations and communities linked through food, hutments and shelter. Together with the abiotic elements of the environment such as substratum, water, light, atmospheric gases, chemicals in solution, etc. the animal/plant associations form almost self-sufficient units called ecosystems. Major ecosystems are the seas, together with estuaries and shores, fresh waters both standing (ponds, lakes) and running (streams, rivers), marshes, deserts, tundras, taiga grasslands and forests. Each ecosystem has its characteristic plant and animal species, often dominated by a few species occurring in large numbers but with equally typical associations of species present in greater variety and smaller numbers. The ecosystem thus comprises the culmination of the morphological and physiological adaptations of its species to their abiotic and biotic environments.

It might be thought that the numbers of species and of individuals in any habitat would remain relatively constant from year to year, maintaining a more or less stable balance. But this is not so. Long-term climatic changes can alter the balance, favouring the development of some species and eliminating others. Developmental or evolutionary changes in the habitats themselves can modify also the original stability. Lakes, for example, tend to work towards their own extinction by filling in with materials brought down by streams and rivers or blown in from the surrounding banks, together with the accumulation of the organic remains of plants and animals. The lake becomes a pond or swamp and progresses eventually to moorland or woodland according to the conditions. Naturally such developmental changes imply equally profound alterations in the flora and fauna.

Numbers can also fluctuate, sometimes between wide limits, even within the context of an apparently stable ecosystem. In some species, the fluctuations may be more or less cyclic. In others, the variations can be very erratic, occurring sporadically with intervening periods of relative stability. Dramatic increases in numbers seldom persist for very long; the original level, perhaps with some overshoot, is re-attained after a comparatively short time. This suggests that the increases are controlled in some way, and provides a clue to the regulation of numbers which maintains the optimum balance of species in an ecosystem.

It is not difficult to appreciate how some of the controls may operate. As numbers increase, the available food supply will become inadequate and more and more individuals will starve. Man's stored food and some of his organic wastes have allowed the growth of large populations of animals such as rodents, gulls and insects which were limited previously by the availability of food. Predators of the species will also increase in numbers because of the initial surplus of prey. With increasing density, endemic diseases can become epidemic. Starvation, predation and disease thus all serve to control population numbers, and by their operation alone or together regulate the balance of species in the environment. More subtle intraspecific effects such as, for example, behavioural changes controlled by population density, can act also as fine adjustments to the major regulators. For a particular species, therefore, a given environment will have an optimum carrying capacity in terms of numbers of individuals related closely to the available food and space.

Man may interfere unwittingly with some of the controls which operate normally within ecosystems. For example, the eradication of particular pests may encourage unnaturally rapid population expansions in other species. Physical disruption of the terrain resulting from large-scale felling of trees, flooding of valleys, canal building, the building of motorways, defoliation methods employed in modern warfare and the laying of surface oil pipes, so alter the environment to provide on the one hand, accelerated routes for migration or dispersal, whilst on the other hand providing impediments to free movement.

The greater the variety and number of species in an ecosystem, the greater will be the number of possible interrelationships. When every ecological niche is occupied, the ecosystem itself will have great stability since the major and minor regulators will be operating at maximum efficiency. Complexity confers stability. In simpler systems, such as those in newly formed lakes, or the artificial associations produced by human agricultural activities, instability is inherent and numbers can fluctuate wildly unless controls other than the natural regulators are brought into play. Similarly, when a species comes to occupy a new environment, either because a niche was previously vacant or because of more successful competition with the current occupier, its numbers will increase until the optimum carrying capacity is reached. If the new environment lacks regulators characteristic of the old, particular predators or diseases, for example, numbers will increase rapidly. The time taken for the population to double itself is a useful measure of such increase. If food and space set the only limits on the carrying capacity of the environment, then when the population is at half the carrying capacity, one more doubling interval reaches the limits and further increases bring the regulators into operation. Without initial restraints, population doubling times can be very short as when rabbits were introduced into Australia, or when insect pests are transported to regions where their natural predators are absent and the abiotic components of their new environments may be more favourable than those of the old.

Starvation, predation, disease and subtle intra- and inter-specific effects serve

masked by another change of atmospheric composition. The burden of dust and aerosol particles carried by the atmosphere have a sunlight-obscuring effect and this more than offsets the heat-trapping of the extra carbon dioxide.

It is interesting that much of the increased turbidity in the atmosphere is of plant origin. The increase in carbon dioxide content has shifted the photosynthetic equilibrium in favour of increased plant growth. Photographs taken from satellites have shown that industrial regions in North America and Western Europe contribute much less to the atmospheric haze (turbidity) than do tropical forests. Vegetative growth produces the release of terpenes, ammonia and hydrogen sulphide; the precursors of aerosols. Desert areas contribute also to the turbidity in the form of fine soil particles. It appears that the outlook, as far as global climatic changes, is not as gloomy as may have appeared at one time. The production of the haze-forming substances may be one of the homeostatic mechanisms operating in the biosphere to provide temperature stabilization.

The problem of scale arises also when effluents containing suspended solids are directed into running waters. Such effluents come from the washings of coal, and from other mining and quarrying processes, from the wood and textile industries, and from the washings of root crops. When passed into lakes in moderate amounts, suspended solids may have little effect upon the bottom fauna, which are adapted to dealing with a continuous rain of detritus from above. Similarly, when discharged into sluggish rivers the effects of the solids may not be disastrous, since some silting is a normal feature of the habitat. But if present in larger amount, the solids can fill the spaces between stones, depriving cryptic species of their normal habitats. Sediment can also cover the surfaces of stones and the holdfasts of the stone fauna become ineffective. Burrowers and tube-dwellers can survive, so at the least a population change is induced. But if the solids do not settle readily, either because they are divided finely or because the water flow is turbulent, then light cannot penetrate the water and plants are unable to survive. Thus except for a few species which depend upon detritus which falls into the water from the banks, the aquatic organisms are eliminated. Once again, the degree of pollution by suspended solids is of importance relative to the conditions in determining whether population change is induced or whether complete disruption of the ecosystem occurs.

Many industrial and sewage effluents may be warmer than the waters into which they are discharged. In general, heat enhances the other pollutional effects —in organic effluents it can reduce the lengths of the biological zones because the organic materials are broken down more rapidly. But heat pollution can also be a product of the operation of nuclear and other power stations, and also of some kinds of industrial processing. In some ways, heat pollution can be considered natural, since hot springs with well-defined biotic communities are typical of some parts of the world. Where water temperatures are increased by only one or two degrees, the effects upon the fauna can be favourable—accelerating maturation rates and reproductive performances. But where animals are adapted to annual periods of low temperatures, increased water temperatures can interfere drastically with their life-cycles, preventing the onset of dormancy for example, so that individuals are active when suitable food is unavailable. High temperatures, of course, will eliminate all animal life, although when the dilution effects are great—when seas or lakes or large rivers are used for cooling—temperatures are unlikely to reach such levels. Changes in population are thus the most likely results of heat pollution.

Although the environment can cope with 'natural' pollutants, at least on the small scale, other pollutants must be regarded strictly as environmental poisons since they have deleterious effects even in small quantities. These poisons can be the waste products of industrial processes such as cyanides, alkalis and acids, tar-acids, phenols and heavy metals; they can be the products of the modern 'developed' society, such as carbon monoxide and lead from motor fuels; or they can be produced deliberately for a specific purpose but prove more widespread in their effects, such as modern synthetic insecticides.

Poisons attract attention because they can affect human beings themselves, and are less subtle in their effects upon the environment than many of the pollutants already discussed. Cyanide waste can kill animals on land and in water, but its possible leakage into drinking water systems arouses most concern. The relationship between accumulated lead and mental health is a problem of modern city life, and although the lead content of the south polar ice sheets, originating from lead alkyls in petrol, has increased dramatically since about 1940, little is known of the effects the wide distribution of lead may have on major ecosystems. Heavy contamination with lead and mercury, together with insecticide residues, may have contributed to the mass deaths of seabirds in the Irish Sea in 1969.

The widespread use of modern synthetic insect pesticides has created serious problems of environmental pollution. The chlorinated hydrocarbons such as DDT, Aldrin, BHC, Dieldrin and Heptachlor are potent insect stomach and contact poisons. They are very persistent—and therefore favoured by agriculturalists since the number of applications for any crop is reduced. But their persistence provides their major environmental disadvantages—the insecticides and their residues can destroy beneficial insects in addition to the pests. The result is that normal associations are broken down, and more and more insecticides are needed to control a specific pest. Moreover, with the elimination of the normal regulators, insects which were not previously considered to be pests can increase in numbers and begin to cause serious damage. Another consequence of insecticide persistence is that of developing immunity to the chemicals by the specific insects which are the targets for the pesticides. The organophosphorus insecticides such as parathion, diazinon, malathion and schradan are very much less persistent than the organochlorines, but suffer from the disadvantage that many of them are highly toxic to mammals, including man, and great care has to be exercised in their application.

Although the drift from insecticide sprays and dusts can be controlled by limiting operations to the appropriate wind and other conditions, so that lethal

Further reading list

1. *Zoophysiology and Ecology*. **1.** Endocrines and Osmoregulation: A Comparative Account of the Regulation of Water and Salt in Vertebrates. P.J. Bentley; Springer-Verlag, 1971.
2. *Transporting Epithelia*. M.J. Berridge and J.L. Oschman; Academic Press, 1972.
3. *Division of Labor in Cells*. G.H. Bourne; Academic Press, 1964.
4. *Pheromones*. M.C. Birch (Ed.); North-Holland Publishing Co., 1974.
5. *The Physiological Clock*. E. Bünning; Heidelberg Science Library, Springer-Verlag, 1967.
6. *Photoperiodism and Seasonal Development of Insects*. A.S. Danilevskii; Oliver and Boyd, 1965.
7. *Mammalian Neuroendocrinology*. B.T. Donovan; McGraw–Hill, 1970.
8. *An Introduction to General and Comparative Physiology*. E. Florey; Saunders & Co., 1966.
9. *The Comparative Endocrinology of the Invertebrates*. K.C. Highnam and L. Hill; Edward Arnold, 1969.
10. *General and Comparative Physiology*. W.S. Hoar; Prentice Hall, 1966.
11. *Principles of Biological Control*. D.F. Horrobin; Medical and Technical Publishing Co. Ltd., 1970.
12. *Animal Hormones*, Parts 1 (1962) and 2 (1970). P.M. Jenkin; Pergamon Press (Oxford).
13. *Adaptation to Desert Environment*. J.P. Kirmiz; Butterworths, 1962.
14. *Animal Body Fluids and their Regulation*. A.P.M. Lockwood; Heinemann, 1963.
15. *The Membranes of Animal Cells*. A.P.M. Lockwood; Edward Arnold, 1971.
16. *Animal Photoperiodism*. B. Lofts; Edward Arnold, 1970.
17. *Mechanisms of Animal Behaviour*. P.R. Marler and W.J. Hamilton III; J. Wiley, 1966.
18. *The Biology of the Cell Cycle*. J.M. Mitchison; Cambridge University Press, 1971.
19. *The Control of Water Balance by the Kidney*. D.B. Moffat; Oxford Biology Readers (Eds J.J. Head and O.E. Lowenstein), 1971.

20. *The Mammalian Heart*. A.R. Muir; Oxford Biology Readers (Eds J.J. Head and O.E. Lowenstein), 1971.
21. *Osmotic and Ionic Regulation in Animals*. W.T.W. Potts and G. Parry; Pergamon Press, 1964.
22. *Ecology*. R.E. Ricklefs; Nelson and Sons, 1973.
23. *Neuroendocrinology*. E. Scharrer and B. Scharrer; Columbia University Press, 1963.
24. *Animal Physiology* (3rd Edition). K. Schmidt-Nielsen; Prentice Hall, 1970.
25. *The Integument: A Textbook of Skin Biology*. R.I.C. Spearman; Cambridge University Press, 1973.
26. The physiology of absorption from the alimentary canal in insects. *Viewpoints in Biology*, Vol. 1, Chapter 5, pages 201–241. J.E. Treherne, 1962.
27. *Life of Marsupials*. H. Tyndale-Biscoe; Edward Arnold, 1973.
28. *The Animal and the Environment*. F.J. Vernberg and W.B. Vernberg; Holt, Rinehart and Winston, 1970.
29. *Colour Change Mechanisms of Cold Blooded Vertebrates*. H. Waring; Academic Press, 1963.
30. *Insect Hormones*. V.B. Wigglesworth; Oliver and Boyd, 1970.
31. *Handbook of Physiology*. Section 4. Adaptations to the Environment. American Physiological Society, 1964.
32. The Current Status of Fish Endocrine Systems. *American Zoologist*, Vol. 13, No. 3, 1973.
33. *Reproduction in Mammals, No. 3: Hormones in Reproduction*. (Eds C.R. Austin and R.V. Short); Cambridge University Press, 1972.
34. *Reproduction in Mammals, No. 4: Reproductive Patterns*. (Eds C.R. Austin and R.V. Short); Cambridge University Press, 1972.
35. *Hormones and the Environment. Memoirs of the Society for Endocrinology, No. 18*. (Eds G.K. Benson and J.G. Phillips); Cambridge University Press, 1970.
36. *Philosophical Transactions of the Royal Society of London. B. Biological Sciences*. A Discussion on Active Transport of Salts and Water in Living Tissues; Vol. 262, pages 83–342, 1971.
37. *Vertebrate Adaptations*. Readings from Scientific American. W.H. Freeman and Co., 1968.
38. The Effects of Pressure on Organisms. *Symposia of the Society for Experimental Biology, No. 26*. (Eds. M.A. Sleigh and A.G. MacDonald); Cambridge University Press, 1972.
39. Nervous and Hormonal Mechanisms of Integration. *Society for Experimental Biology Symposia, No. 20*. (Ed. G.M. Hughes); Cambridge University Press, 1966.
40. Dormancy and Survival. *Symposia of the Society for Experimental Biology, No. 23*. (Ed. H.W. Woolhouse); Cambridge University Press, 1969.